Never to Be a Mother

Never to Be a Mother

A Guide for All Women Who Didn't—or Couldn't—Have Children

Linda Hunt Anton

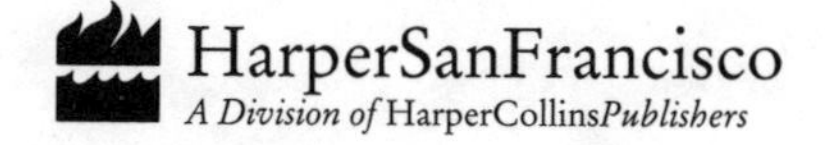
HarperSanFrancisco
A Division of HarperCollins*Publishers*

 For information address HarperCollins Publishers, 10 East 53rd Street, New York, NY 10022.

Text design by Adriane Bosworth.

FIRST EDITION

Library of Congress Cataloging-in-Publication Data

Anton, Linda Hunt.
Never to be a mother : a guide for all women who didn't—or couldn't—have children / Linda Hunt Anton — 1st ed.
p. cm.
Includes bibliographical references (p. 187) and index.
ISBN 0-06-250079-1 (alk. paper)
1. Childlessness—United States—Psychological aspects.
2. Infertility—United States—Psychological aspects. I. Title.
HQ536.A63 1992 91–58137
306.87—dc20 CIP

---

92 93 94 95 96 ❖ RRD(H) 10 9 8 7 6 5 4 3 2 1

This edition is printed on acid-free paper that meets the American National Standards Institute Z39.48 Standard.

This book is dedicated to my husband John, who would have been Jenny's father.

Contents

PART THREE

TEN STEPS TO RESOLUTION 61

PART FOUR

STARTING A SELF-HELP GROUP 179

Preface

Nearly one-third of my life, more than fifteen years, has been touched by the sadness and loss of being childless.

I no longer remember if I always assumed I would be a mother. Having grown up in a small Mormon community in southern Utah, I imagine the assumption was always there. All the adult women in my life—mother, grandmothers, aunts, neighbors, family friends—were homemakers, and all (with a few exceptions) were mothers. That is what women did; they married and raised a family.

Although my early memories of wanting a child are hazy, I know exactly when the subject became an emotional one for me—as I approached the age of thirty. Exploring the world beyond my hometown had filled the years after high school with challenge and excitement: four years at Utah State University, two years at the Graduate School of Social Work at the University of Washington, marriage (to a man who had two children by a previous marriage), a move to San Francisco, several years working in England. I was content with my life—until I approached thirty.

Now it is commonplace for women over thirty to have children; when I was that age it was not. First pregnancies after age thirty were considered risky for both mother and fetus. As I neared my thirtieth birthday, I felt a growing urgency to start a family. I wanted a baby, and time was slipping by. My husband was ambivalent. He had been hurt by the loss of his children through divorce, and he feared being hurt again. Because we had always relied on two incomes, he worried too about our financial situation.

I thought that I could live a good life without a child if I had to. After all, I had done so for many years already. Unlike my two sisters—the older had five children at the time, and the younger had two (and would later have three more)—my adult years had not revolved around children. I loved my work as a social worker, enjoyed traveling, and had many interests. I thought I could adjust to being childless if I had to, but I needed a decision. I could not keep wanting and hoping for a baby if there would be no baby because of my husband's ambivalence. I had to know which way to guide my heart. "Of course we'll have children, but this isn't the right time" became my husband's refrain. I reacted with anger, tears, and resentment, but I yielded to his indecision. Soon we had settled into a broken-record routine on the subject; this routine lasted the remaining ten years of our marriage.

Many years after our divorce, while I was in therapy, I came to see that I had inadvertently played a part in my childlessness. Because I did not know how, because I was not strong enough then to value my needs as much as my husband's, I had turned the final decision over to him.

When I married my present husband, a very different kind of man, he welcomed another family even though he had two grown daughters. He was as excited at the prospect of a baby as I was. He wanted to be the father of my Jenny, the little girl I had dreamed of all those years.

When I did not get pregnant right away, I consulted a local gynecologist, who recommended that I keep a basal-body-temperature chart. I conscientiously took my temperature every morning; we timed intercourse religiously to coincide with ovulation. The start of each period brought disappointment; the passing months brought ever-greater anxiety. We had joined the roller-coaster ride of ups and downs so familiar to infertile couples.

At my urging, the doctor finally agreed that the charts were not enough. He recommended a tubal insufflation test, in which carbon dioxide gas is blown into the uterus through a tube inserted into the cervical canal. The test not only helps determine if the fallopian tubes are open but also aids in conception because it helps clear minor obstructions from the tubes. "Most of my patients get pregnant after the test," he informed me, and throughout the painful procedure I clung to his words. I would submit to any procedure, no matter how painful, to get pregnant. The test results looked promising, the tubes seemed to be open, and my hopes soared. But the months went by and I did not get pregnant, and soon the doctor lost interest in my situation. After all, as he pointed out, I was over forty. Yes! I did not need him to tell me that my time was running out! Already I had wasted almost a precious year.

After intense searching I finally located a fertility specialist I liked and trusted, but he was leaving on vacation. I could hardly tolerate the one-month delay; it was unbearable to waste even one more day. But I waited. Within a week of his return I was in the hospital. In the course of the preliminary physical exam, he had discovered a mass that he thought might be cancer; surgery was imperative.

When the doctor gave me the preoperative papers to sign, papers that gave him permission to perform a hysterectomy if necessary, I stared at them numbly. I did not want to sign. I couldn't. I wouldn't. Every part of me screamed, "No!" But I signed.

Two days later, sick with apprehension, I went into surgery. Would I wake to learn I had cancer? Would I wake to learn I had no uterus? I do not know which I dreaded more.

I did not have cancer; the mass was endometriosis. Thanks to the doctor's understanding of what a child meant to me and his willingness to help give me that chance, I emerged from surgery with ovaries and uterus intact. He had spent five hours removing the endometriosis, which adhered to one ovary and other organs.

Then followed several years of infertility workups. Tests showed that my husband had no problems, so diagnostic procedures focused on me. Each month I went to a medical laboratory, where blood was drawn and analyzed to check estrogen and progesterone levels as a way to determine my pattern of ovulation. Irregular ovulation, probably due to early menopause, was detected, and Clomid was prescribed to regulate it.

I hate to remember those years—the tears, the sadness, the sorrow, the dreams at night of holding a baby, only to wake to empty arms. Grocery shopping became an ordeal; I could not bear to see the mothers with their babies and little children. Throughout it all my husband shared my pain, tried to comfort me, experienced his own loss.

And then another surgery, a laparoscopy, which enables the physician to visually inspect the fallopian tubes. When my doctor told me, as kindly as he could, that both tubes now had major blockage, that although it was not impossible that I would conceive, it was unlikely, I knew I had reached the end of the line. "Enough!" I cried to myself. "I must face the fact that I will never have a child, that I will never be a mother." I knew that as long as I had hope, I would have pain, and I decided to call an end to both. I never considered adoption. Adoption meant years of waiting, years of searching, with no guarantee of a child, and I could bear no more disappointment.

I forced myself, rather severely I think now, to say to myself every day, "You will never be a mother! You will never have a child! Accept it and get on with your life!" I would not talk about my feelings, not even to my husband. When he broached the subject, I would say abruptly, "It's not going to happen. That's the way it is. I don't want to talk about it."

Then gradually, as time passed, I allowed my sorrow to surface. I let my Jenny die, and I mourned her loss. I went into therapy and learned to understand and forgive myself for the part I had played in my earlier childlessness. I was determined *not* to let childlessness ruin my life, and eventually, largely through sheer determination, I found my path to resolution.

This book originated—although I did not know it at the time—during those dark days when I first acknowledged that I would never have a child. In the past I had found guidance and consolation in self-help books that dealt with other issues. Assuming there would be a book that could help me accept my permanent childlessness, I went to a large bookstore in downtown San Francisco. My search through the women's and psychology sections yielded nothing, but I did not want to ask the clerk for help. When I could not even yet talk about my feelings to my mother, my sister, my best friends, how could I say to a stranger, "I need a book that can help me accept that I'll never have a child"?

When a young male clerk approached and asked if he could help, I flushed. I felt as though a *B* blazed on my chest: *B* as in *Barren.* I stammered out what I wanted, not quite in a whisper, but as discreetly as possible. Soon two clerks were discussing my request—in everyday tones that other people could hear!—and I fought back tears of humiliation as the clerk led me to the section of infertility books. But I had already read infertility books, including chapters on the emotional impact of infertility and alternative ways to become a parent. I would *never* be a parent. That was *not* what I needed. I fled the bookstore having found no book, no help. Years later, after much healing had taken place, I decided to write the book I had needed earlier. I knew other women must need it too.

My story has a happy postscript. Although I am not a mother, I am a grandmother. Several years ago one of my nieces who lives near me told me she was pregnant and asked if I would be the baby's grandmother, because her own mother, my sister, had died. I was ecstatic. Being present at the birth of her daughter, my first grandchild, was one of the most moving experiences of my life. A year and a half later one of my stepdaughters gave birth to a baby girl, and this time my husband and I shared the joy of seeing his first and my second grandchild arrive. Now I have a grandson too, my niece's second child, and I am unabashedly playing the grandmother role for all it is worth.

During my years of social work practice I had done extensive therapy with women—individually, in groups, and as part of family therapy. I knew that mothering was an inextricable part of many women's feminine identity. How, I began to wonder, had other childless women resolved the incongruity between their vision of themselves, which included being a mother, and their reality, which did not? What, if any, had been their paths to resolution?

One of the first steps I took to find the answer was to place notices in one local and three national publications. The notice read:

> Childless? Therapist studying emotional impact of childlessness on women who wanted children seeks contact with women resigned to childlessness.

Another step was to write to the many childless women I knew in my own circle: relatives, friends, daughters of friends, former colleagues, any women I knew personally who I *thought* might have wanted children. I explained my project and asked if the women would be interested and willing to participate. (A copy of the questionnaire that guided face-to-face and telephone interviews and that was mailed to women who could not be interviewed directly is at the end of this book.)

A diverse group of women from across the country participated. Ages ranged from twenty-four to seventy-eight. Educational backgrounds varied from high school to medical school education. Some women were homemakers; others worked outside the home. A few participants had never had a significant relationship with a man, others had had intense relationships but had never married, and still others were married, divorced, or widowed. Their reactions to childlessness varied from intense distress to mild disappointment.

The individual women you will read about in the book are composites of the many women I interviewed. I present the women in this fashion both to protect the identity of each woman and to convey as succinctly as possible the common experiences and feelings of many women.

The generous and uninhibited sharing of these women constitutes the lifeblood of this book. What I learned from them touched me deeply. Their stories—their dreams, their sorrows, their struggles, their healing processes, and their varying degrees of resolution—were powerful beyond anything I had anticipated. This book is our contribution, mine and theirs, to all the women who want to live a rich, full, happy life, even if it must be a life without children.

Acknowledgments

From the bottom of *my* heart, I thank all the childless women who opened *their* hearts to me. The generosity with which they shared their experiences and feelings touched me deeply. I learned from them, and we learned together, about the far-reaching impact childlessness has on the lives of women who want children. Their stories give the book life; their contribution has been invaluable.

Three friends who are writers are gratefully acknowledged: Madelon Phillips and J. Renee Gilbert offered tremendous support and encouragement during the writing of the book, and they read and critiqued the entire manuscript as it evolved. With great generosity of spirit, they also sent roses when they learned the book was going to be published. Elizabeth Holmes read an early draft and helped steer me in a more coherent direction when I needed help with that.

I thank my two friends Kathleen Keady and Marian Cole, who willingly read and discussed the manuscript. The feedback from them, as childless women, is greatly appreciated, as are their affection and support.

I am deeply grateful to Barbara Moulton, my editor at HarperSanFrancisco. She had the foresight to see the need for this book, and her excitement for it never wavered. She also deserves credit for the book's final form. It was she who suggested that the information on resolution be organized into a ten-step program, a format that makes the material more accessible and helpful to the reader. I am also grateful to the many other staff at HarperSanFrancisco who enthusiastically embraced the book.

And I thank my husband John for his interest, support, and help. He also read the manuscript as it evolved, and he brought his disciplined, logical mind to bear on it. Where there was vagueness, he asked for clarity. Where there was psychological jargon, he asked for understandable language. When I was discouraged, he cheered me on. He knows what it means to me to be childless; he believes in the book as much as I do.

The stories in this book accurately reflect the feelings, experiences, and circumstances expressed by the women interviewed by the author, but all names, locations, and identifying details have been changed.

Who This Book Is About and For

THE CHILDLESS WOMEN THIS BOOK ADDRESSES

If you are a woman who wanted to be a mother, who wanted to have children, but never will, this book is for you. Permanent childlessness crosses all religious, racial, ethnic, educational, and socioeconomic lines. In all times and all places, women who wanted children have had to face permanent childlessness.

When most people think of childless women, they think of infertile married women, and in this age, when medical miracles such as fertility drugs, in vitro fertilization, insemination, and embryo transplantation are trumpeted daily in the news, an even greater poignancy is felt by the infertile women whose childless state will not be changed by the new scientific advancements. But they are not the only ones who will never be mothers.

Many single women also long for children, as do women with medical problems or physical or mental handicaps. Women who love men who already have children and do not want more must choose between the men they love and their unborn children. Some women caught in destructive relationships refrain from having children because they know they could not provide a home environment conducive to a child's growth and development. Lesbian women, until recently, rarely had children. Religious women who devote their lives to God may long for a child of their own. There are many paths to childlessness.

THE WOMEN THIS BOOK DOES NOT ADDRESS

Some women become mothers through adoption. In many ways their experiences parallel those of the childless women this book is about. Their longings and frustrations are the same before they adopt a child, and some women continue to long for a biological child even after they adopt. But while there are similarities between the two groups, there is one profound difference. Women who adopt *do* become mothers; they *do* have children.

When I use the phrase *childless women,* I mean women who are permanently childless.

Other women deliberately choose *not* to have children. They *do not* want to be mothers. But they are not the childless women of whom I write. *When I refer in this book to childless women, I mean women who wanted children. I automatically exclude women who did not want children.* Motherhood can be a rich and rewarding experience, but it is not the only way women create full, satisfactory lives for themselves. Women who choose not to have children experience their childlessness differently than do women who want children. The former have the life they choose (in that respect at least) and can appreciate the advantages of *childfree living;* the latter must contend with their second choice, not having children.

CHILDLESS MEN

This book's focus on childless women in no way suggests that childless men who want to be fathers long less intensely for a child or suffer less from their unfulfilled dreams. They too experience loss and disappointment. But because women's traditional roles have been defined as wife and mother, while men's primary role has been defined as provider, the meaning of childlessness *does* differ for men and women. Childlessness strikes at the heart, the essence of a woman's identity. Men who want children may also need help resolving their loss, and I hope some of the ideas in this book will help them. But since I am a childless woman and I identify with a woman's experience, it is to childless women that I speak.

Never to Be a Mother

PART ONE

The Loss

The dream of having children, of being a mother is a dream that lies deep within the heart. Women who want children cherish the dream, nurture it, believe it will come true one day. But not all dreams come true. When the dream of having children dies, when at last it is laid to rest, childless women still experience loss that is deep and lasting. If you have ever said or thought, "I will never have a child; I will never be a mother," you know how profound the loss can be. At times it feels unbearable.

Although many people associate loss with prior possession, as when a loved one dies, loss also occurs when there is a failure to obtain that which the heart desires. Because this loss—the longing for that which will never be—is less tangible, less visible, it may be overlooked or minimized, but it is real nonetheless.

The loss is real because the children who live in our hearts are real. We *see* them in our mind's eye. We know what they look like: whether they have light or dark hair, whether they are girls or boys. And we see ourselves as mothers. We picture ourselves holding a baby, nursing it, bathing it. We see ourselves combing a daughter's hair, teaching a son to read, taking our children to the beach. Some women *feel* like mothers, mothers without children.

HIDDEN LOSS, SILENT PAIN

"Give me children, or else I die!" Rachel cried in Genesis 30:1. Like Rachel, some women cry their anguish to the world. The anger and tears of their despair are apparent to everyone around them. Most childless women, however, display no evidence of their disappointment and sadness as they go about the business of living their daily lives. Their loss is not verbalized or shared, even with close friends or family. It is silent, hidden from all but the women who experience it.

Many women feel too vulnerable to share their feelings with others. I was such a woman. In other matters I shared my disappointments, frustrations, and sorrows quite readily with family and friends. When my sister died, when I went through a divorce, I cried, I raged, *and* I turned to important people in my life for support and help. Not so when I experienced the worst of my sorrow about not having children; then I could turn only to my husband. No one else knew that I woke from baby dreams and cried for hours afterward. I told no one else how I dreaded grocery shopping because my heart ached when I saw other women pushing children in grocery carts. I felt too vulnerable, too tender to expose myself.

Of course not every feeling, every aspect of our lives must be shared with others. Too often, though, when we suffer in silence, we cut ourselves off from the comfort and support of others who care. They may wonder if we wanted children, wonder if we are disappointed not to have them, but, sensing how sensitive the subject is, they hold back, not wanting to be intrusive or rude. Permanent childlessness is discussed so rarely in our society that it has taken on an almost taboo quality. Neither the woman nor those who care about her feel comfortable broaching the subject.

The Enduring Impact

Few people realize how long childlessness remains an issue in a woman's life. It may intrude as a sensitive issue for fifteen to twenty years. It may last even longer, a lifetime, as a hovering presence around the edges of your life. Women I interviewed in their seventies still have passing sadness about not having had children and grandchildren. Women in their fifties remember how many children they wanted and often remember the names they had chosen. I realized when I was writing this book that nearly one-third of my life had been touched by the sadness of being childless. Given how long permanent childlessness remains an issue in many women's lives, it is surprising that so little attention has been paid to this important issue; it is surprising that so little help is available.

The Assumption of Motherhood

It is *not* surprising that childlessness has an intense, enduring impact on our lives, given that mothering and female identity are inextricably linked from a very early age. For centuries, women's primary roles have been defined as those of wife and mother. Even today, a woman who chooses *not* to have a child is considered abnormal by many people. Adult women *are* mothers—that is the norm. (A number of women I interviewed had rebelled against the assumption that all women will be mothers. The women's movement has brought a heightened awareness of the pressure our paternalistic society exerts on women to be mothers, and these women were determined *not* to be pushed into the old mold. They were therefore astonished—and amused—at the unexpected and powerful need *they* felt to have a child, usually when they reached their thirties, a biological and psychological need that had nothing to do with society's expectations.)

Most of us, however, always assumed as girls and young women that we would be mothers. Many of us went beyond assumption—we *knew* we wanted to be mothers. Some of us articulated it as a goal, perhaps our most important life goal.

From the time we are little girls, most females cherish the dream of one day being a mother, with babies and children of our own. As children we mother our dolls, feed them, rock them to sleep, scold them. As teens and young women we dream of falling in love, marrying, and having a family. As we proceed blithely through adolescence and young adulthood, the possibility of being childless never enters our minds. We believe that when we are ready, at a time of our choosing, we will have our children.

Reality Intrudes

Reality intrudes in many ways. Sometimes it slips in slowly, softly, with the passing years. Single women, confident at first that they will marry and have children, begin to wonder as the years go by. "There's still time," they assure themselves as they approach their late twenties. When they reach their middle to late thirties, hope fades, and they begin to accept their reality. They say, "Maybe it isn't going to happen for me." For them, awareness dawns gradually over many years.

At times reality strikes abruptly. A sudden hysterectomy, a diagnosis of congenital sterility, or a ruptured ectopic pregnancy leaves the woman reeling. She has no time to consider, let alone assimilate, the possibility of being childless before she is hit with the certainty that she will never give birth to a child.

Other times reality provides the roller-coaster ride so familiar to women with infertility problems. They (and their partners) soar to heights of hope and excitement, then plunge to depths of frustration and despair, as promising new drugs, new procedures, new treatments are tried and fail, and each month the unwelcome menstrual cycle starts. Women who have no difficulty getting pregnant but who miscarry repeatedly also experience emotional highs and lows. Each new pregnancy brings hope that *this* one will be carried to term; each miscarriage brings disappointment.

DIFFERENT EXPERIENCE

Childlessness is not the same experience for every woman. Your reaction, your experience of loss will be unique in many ways, determined by the complex social, psychological, and family influences that have helped shape you into the person you are today. In many other ways your experiences and feelings will be like those of other childless women.

The first woman I interviewed, a seventy-eight-year-old friend of mine, started the interview by saying, "I wanted children, but I was never one of the frantic ones." I knew immediately what she meant, because I had been one of the frantic ones. Although it is a simplistic division, most women do fall into one of two categories. Either they experienced their childlessness as traumatic and for a period of their lives felt frantic about the issue, or they did not. If you feel that your life will be meaningless unless you are a mother, you may well be devastated at the prospect of never having a child. If you have always thought you would like to be a mother but know you can have a fulfilling life without children, you may react with passing wistfulness. Reactions range along a continuum from mild disappointment to intense grief.

The experience of childlessness not only differs for each woman but also is experienced differently by the same woman at different times in her life. Age, marital status, and satisfaction with career and life in general are influential factors. A woman in her early to middle twenties who wants children may be fully satisfied with her young adult life—a new career, her own apartment, travel, romances, new friends. She will have her children later. When that same woman approaches thirty-five with no child in sight, she may feel the beginnings of concern or even panic because she knows her biological time clock is running out. In her late thirties and early forties she may experience intense disappointment, loss, even depression. In her fifties and sixties childlessness may fade as an issue as she finds fulfillment through other relationships and enjoys the freedom to develop and explore new parts of herself. As old age nears, the picture may change yet again. The loss of a partner, the loss of friends, may reawaken feelings of not being vital to anyone. She may long again for children—and now grandchildren too—who would alleviate the emptiness and loneliness of her life.

When Childlessness Is Traumatic

If you *were* emotionally traumatized by your childlessness, the experience may have shaken the foundation of your life. Intense feelings of despair, anger, guilt, shame, self-pity, envy, and jealousy are not uncommon. Many women frequently experience mild or severe depression.

Years ago I saw a statue in the Dutch city of Rotterdam that I remember still. As the title, *Monument to a Devastated City,* suggests, Rotterdam was devastated by bombing during the Second World War. The statue is a larger-than-life human figure that twists and writhes in pain, arms raised to the heavens. A gaping hole lies at the center of the figure where the vital organs should be. For many of us, for part of our lives, that is how we feel about being childless.

The women I interviewed spoke and wrote eloquently of their feelings, and in the next six sections, which focus on reactions to childlessness, I have used their words. Remember, as you read, that the feelings expressed are often irrational.

On Sadness and Despair

- "Sometimes the pain is overwhelming, and it becomes very physical. Your heart hurts. The hardest part is just a feeling of loneliness. Maybe a feeling of not being whole. I don't know, maybe like having a twin sister that you know should be there but isn't."
- "In many ways I think my general hopelessness and disappointment with life generate from childlessness. The feeling of not being vital to anyone is very big with me."
- "It's been very hard for me to deal with. I cry a lot, feel sorry for myself. I feel like no one understands how I feel. It's like being in a room full of people and you're still alone. The pain for me is still real every time I see somebody with a baby. I cry for what will never be."
- "They say time heals all wounds, but I think this is one wound that will never heal, no matter how much time passes. Sometimes I try to convince myself that I am glad I'm childless, but who am I fooling? Myself. There will always be that empty space."
- "I feel empty inside; I feel alone. I mourn. I have even felt suicidal. It's a pain that doesn't go away."

- "When I became aware of my infertility, depression set in. It set in deeply, and I didn't share it with anyone, not even my husband. I had a nervous breakdown. I had an affair because I thought maybe I could get pregnant with another man. I also was addicted to smoking some very potent marijuana. I was a mess. I really went to hell and back."
- "The pain passes; the loss is forever."
- "There isn't anything I want to go past fifty for. That whole excitement, the hope for the future. I'll never feel that again. Not like I did when I was pregnant."
- "Not being able to have a child has shaken my belief about life and the world. I used to believe we could create certain kinds of energy around us; we could help determine what our lives would be. Now that makes no sense. If people who are as loving and gentle and want a child as much as we do can't have children, then the world is an unfair place."

On Guilt and Self-Blame

- "I blamed myself for a long time. I still do, but I try not to, because it's not my fault. At least I tell myself that, but I don't really believe it."
- "It's maybe some God judgment. I don't know. There's got to be an element of that. Maybe the judgment is, 'You aren't a mother because you couldn't have handled it; you wouldn't have been a good mother.' "
- "I went to a body therapist, and he had me talk to the child, because I did see her. I saw the little girl that I would have had. I felt guilt about not having a child. I felt there was a

child who wanted to come into the world, and I somehow was not able to bring that about. I felt there was something wrong with me, that I couldn't give this child what she wanted. I felt like it was abandonment before the fact."

- "I feel like I'm not a complete woman somehow. You're supposed to be able to have children if you're a woman."
- "I'm so abnormal. We are, childless women; we're not normal, and because of that people don't know how to talk to us."
- "You accuse yourself. I feel guilty because every pregnancy ended in a miscarriage, like I must have done something wrong."

On Anger

- "I have a lot of anger, and I don't know what to do with it. I'm angry at the world and the inequity in it. It's so frustrating because there's no one you can direct it at. There's no villain."
- "Sometimes anger will come out against people who have what I don't have."
- "I get so angry when I read about parents who abuse their children or women who abandon newborn babies. Why should they have babies when I can't?!"

On Feeling Robbed

- "I can't help but think a lot of women would feel robbed by nature or whatever that force is. A nonpersonal God or whatever, but you're still ripped off."
- "We are victimized by fate, if you will, or by our own bodies."

On Vulnerability

- "I don't think there's any area that could be more vulnerable. You're talking about your own inner child in some ways."
- "Because it's such a personal thing, you don't manifest it outwardly, and people think you don't experience it. They just take it for granted you don't."
- "I have this great reluctance to open up the sorrow again, even in therapy. I just don't want to do that. I remember dreams as a child about being naked in front of a classroom, and it's comparable, absolute vulnerability when you open to the pain on this subject. I'm never going to be that vulnerable again."

On Shame and Social Discomfort

- "I went to a support group, and what came up for me was a sense of shame. It's somehow as if I'm not a whole person, that not everything is there. So it's shameful. Something to be ashamed of. Something to be hidden. That's what I feel."
- "I hate going to the gynecologist. There are baby pictures everywhere; it's as if every single woman is supposed to have a baby. I can't stand going to get checkups. It's like women are baby factories, and you're a broken part."
- "You walk around, and everything is geared around children. You're in an age group where everybody else is having babies."
- "People think if you don't have children you don't like kids or you're selfish, uncaring, don't want to tie yourself down. They don't ever think that maybe you just can't."

- "I just hate it when people ask, 'How many children do you have?' or 'Don't you want to have children?' "
- "I hated Mother's Day with an absolute passion. I can't even begin to tell you. Mother's Day would come, and my stepchildren would send cards to their biological mother, and I really hated it. It got so bad that one year I actually left home for the day. I couldn't even bear to be home."

Your feelings may be similar to those just described, or they may be different. Each woman's experience is unique. But it is helpful to know that intense feelings of anger, shame, or despair are not unusual.

SIGNIFICANT LOSSES

Loss of Love

If I were to choose one word that is at the heart of the childless woman's experience, that word would be *loss*. And the greatest loss is loss of love: love you would give to your children, love you would receive from your children. To be childless is to lose enduring, unconditional love. Mother love is universally accepted as the most unselfish, powerful love of which humans are capable. The intense bond between mother and child has been recognized by people throughout the ages; artists and theologians have extolled its virtues.

Often the mother-child bond endures longer than any other bond, longer than friendship bonds, longer than many marriage bonds. As one woman said, "Husbands come and go, but children are with you forever." In the early formative years of our lives, our mothers minister to our basic need to feel loved and secure, which is why the mother-child bond comes to symbolize the quintessence of safety and love. The symbolism may be more a matter of fantasy than reality for women whose mothers did not provide love and security, but even these women know that a troubled mother-child bond tends to last throughout life. The mother-child bond may even continue to influence beyond the grave. I think of how often my husband prefaces a remark with, "My mother was a wise woman. She always said . . ." and how often a good friend laughs and says, "My mother used to say to me . . ." I know that often when *I* need a pick-me-up, I will prepare a special dish my mother used to cook, and it *does* make me feel better. Don't we all, when we are ill (and unattended) at home, remember with longing the loving care our mothers once provided? Perhaps the most poignant example of the enduring mother-child bond is found in nursing homes, where confused elderly women search ceaselessly for their mothers.

Loss of Friendship, Loss of Support

Loss of an adult child's friendship is another significant loss, and as we reach middle age we become more aware of this particular loss. Many of us had less-than-satisfactory relationships with our mothers when we were children or adolescents, but as adults, with few exceptions, we do develop an understanding of and appreciation for our mothers. Most of us come to accept that our mothers did the best they could, given who they were and the circumstances of their lives. We learn to count our mothers as friends, and we wish we could look forward to an adult child's friendship.

And we miss more than just friendship. Being childless means one significant supportive network is missing in life. At times of crisis—divorce, unemployment, diagnosis of a life-threatening illness—children and grandchildren are sources of comfort and support. Old age, if we live long enough, brings a diminution of senses, mobility, and physical strength. The old are usually more vulnerable, less active, more likely to be in poor health. Loneliness can be a constant companion. As our parents age and need more care, as we look ahead to our old age, we wonder, "Who will be there for me?" When our parents die, when we lose a partner, we long for the love and support, the network that children and grandchildren provide.

Loss of Continuity

Like all living things, we human beings are subject to nature's inexorable cycle of renewal. We too are of the earth. Just as spring's new growth matures in summer, fades in autumn, dies in winter, and blooms again next spring, so do we begin as babies, grow, develop, mature, age, and die. New babies are born and the cycle continues. We see our place in the continuing cycle when we consider the parents and grandparents and their parents and grandparents who went before us. Women with children see their children, grandchildren, great-grandchildren extending continuously into the future. But the childless woman has no such vision. As she matures, as her parents age and die, she knows the cycle will not continue; it will end with her.

This loss of continuity of generations takes on an even greater poignancy for a childless woman who is adopted. Even though she may dearly love her adoptive parents and siblings, she misses continuity with the family who went before her; she misses continuity with family who would follow her. She lacks blood ties in both directions. As one woman said, "All my life I've longed to know who my biological parents were; I've needed those *roots*. And now, because I don't have children, I've missed a commitment to eternity. I've lost out both ways."

Loss of Experience

Women who wanted children know they have missed one of the most profound, most exacting, most rewarding experiences a woman can have. Bearing children is a natural part of life, and childless women's bodies may ache for the biological experiences of pregnancy, childbirth, and nursing. Their arms and their wombs feel empty when there is no baby to cuddle and love.

Women want the challenge of raising children, of helping them grow from infants into secure, happy, productive human beings. Just as the young girl learns about the world around her and the adolescent girl learns to relate to her peers and find an identity of her own, so the adult woman learns and matures through mothering. Women who cannot test themselves in the demanding role of mother miss an age-appropriate developmental challenge.

TEN STEPS TO RESOLUTION

Although childlessness is often traumatic and the loss deep and lasting, resolution is possible. Resolution means learning to accept a major disappointment in your life. Depending on the intensity of your desire for a child and your concomitant grief, the adjustment required may be similar to the adjustment that follows a crippling illness or accident or the death of a loved one. The adjustments are not in life-style as you have known it but rather in expectations, in how you wanted to live, how you assumed you would live, who you wanted to be.

Resolution is not easy, and it is not inevitable. Women who fail to resolve their feelings sentence themselves to a life of dissatisfaction. One woman who had *not* resolved her pain organized her entire life so as to minimize contact with people who had children; exposure to children was too painful for her.

The heart of this book, Part III, focuses on resolution. The ten steps to resolution that are summarized here will be explored in depth there.

Step 1: Acknowledging and Experiencing the Loss

You have experienced loss. Denying, minimizing, or avoiding your feelings will delay the healing process. Mourning the loss of the child who lived in your imagination and heart, mourning the loss of your identity as a mother, is a painful but necessary step in healing.

Step 2: Understanding the Loss

By identifying the psychological and social factors that shaped you and your wish for a child, you can better understand your unique needs. This helps you deal with feelings that otherwise may seem overwhelming and helps you identify alternative ways to meet those needs.

Step 3: Surviving the Loss

Childlessness does not have to ruin your life. As you find the determination to move beyond loss, you see that you can still influence and create a life of your choosing. You no longer feel like a victim; you start to see yourself as a survivor, one who has overcome disappointment and heartache.

Step 4: Letting Go of Blame

Rational or irrational blame, whether of yourself or others, delays resolution. Identifying the part you may have played, albeit unwittingly, in your childlessness helps you forgive others. Gentleness, kindness, and understanding help you forgive yourself.

Step 5: Talking to Significant Others

When you talk to others who care about you, you receive their understanding and support. You no longer suffer silently. When we tell others what we need from them, they are better able to respond in a caring way.

Step 6: Using Available Resources

By connecting directly with other women who wanted children or by finding childless role models to emulate, you learn how others have coped. Therapy, spiritual or religious pursuits, and support groups can help.

Step 7: Rechanneling Mothering Energy

By broadening your concept of mothering to include other people's children, adults, animals, and the planet, you find ways to redirect and use your powerful nurturing energy.

Step 8: Including Children in Your Life

You do not have to deprive yourself of the pleasure and fun of being with children. There are many ways to have children in your life.

Step 9: Maximizing the Advantages of Childfree Living

Women without children have fewer financial obligations and worries; they have more freedom and time. Learn to appreciate and enjoy the advantages of a *childfree* life.

Step 10: Embracing the Quest for Feminine Wholeness

All women search for meaning in their lives; all need to know who they are beyond the roles they play. By exploring your deepest needs, longings, and hurts, by confronting your beliefs about yourself and about life, you embark on an inward spiritual journey. You learn to value yourself, to feel whole.

Before we look ahead to resolution, however, it is helpful to know where we have been. Part II examines the paths to childlessness, the many and varied reasons why women who wanted children end up childless.

PART TWO

Paths to Childlessness

The paths to childlessness are as many and as varied as the women who travel them. Some paths progress in a straightforward manner from start to finish. Other paths meander and fork. Because the paths can be very different, they may appear unrelated, but all lead to the same childless end.

Not all paths can be described, of course, so I have focused on the most prevalent reasons why women do not have children. Unfortunately, this means that some women, emotionally or developmentally disabled women, to name a few, are not directly addressed, but they too may long to have children. Women whose paths are not described will nonetheless find comfort in the stories retold here; their feelings, their needs, and their longings are addressed, even if their particular situations are not.

SINGLE WOMEN

If you are a single woman who wanted to marry and have children, you may feel that you have lost out twice because you have neither the husband nor the child you desired. Even though single women know that a husband and a child are not guarantees of, or prerequisites for, a happy life, most single women who wanted to experience marriage and motherhood regret missing those experiences. They feel their lives would have been even richer and fuller had they been wives and mothers.

Growing up, finding and marrying the right man, and then having children is the pattern most women expect their lives to follow. Since the natural sequence is seen as marriage and then children, it is marriage, not motherhood, that becomes imbued with urgency when the possibility of remaining single, and childless, first looms. While there are notable exceptions, most single women express primary sadness and disappointment about not marrying. Being childless is a secondary issue.

A single woman is often subjected to pressure, especially in her twenties and early thirties, by well-meaning friends and relatives who ask frequently about marriage plans or prospects. The pressure usually lessens as the woman grows older and others' expectations for her change, though then people may say (when the single woman is not there), "I wonder why she never married," the implication being that there is something wrong with a woman who did not marry. Even though the single woman likes herself, knows she is competent at work, has many friends, many talents, she may make the same judgment. "Why couldn't I sustain a relationship that led to marriage?" "What's wrong with me?" are questions that may nibble away at her self-esteem.

If you are like many of the women I interviewed, you stayed single *because* nothing is wrong with you. These women are single because they are strong individuals, confident and competent enough to be alone. They do not flee into marriage because they fear the alternative. They have (or had) opportunities to marry, but, as one woman says, "The right man never asked me." The potential husbands they have met are not men with whom they wish to spend the rest of their lives, and they refuse to compromise their hopes, their dreams, their lives. They are not willing to marry just to be married, and they are not willing to marry just to have children.

Almost all single women consider single motherhood, either through pregnancy or adoption, and then decide against it. For many women a child is part of a package deal, the package being the traditional family with both father and mother. They need the complete family to satisfy their dreams. Other women reject the stressful, difficult reality, for both mother and child, of single-parent families. They have seen sisters and friends struggle to balance the demands of family and work as the single head of a household; they know the price paid in guilt and exhaustion.

Even though they long to be mothers, most single women *do not* feel traumatized or frantic about being childless. The reason is not that they wanted children less than married women do but rather that they always kept the motherhood-child issue at arm's length. If they had married, childlessness would have been more traumatic, because then being a mother would be no longer a dream but a real possibility.

Nonetheless, as single women see friends their age (and then younger) marry and have children, they are reminded of what is missing in their lives. Attending bridal and baby showers stirs up old longings and becomes an ordeal. Vicarious pleasure in sharing others' joy loses its charm. One woman sums it up when she says, "It's not that I begrudge other women the happiness of a husband and a baby. I just want the same thing for myself."

"A Softer Disappointment"

IRIS'S STORY

Iris, an energetic, ambitious, fifty-four-year-old woman, lives in Washington, D.C. She grew up in a loving, close, Irish Catholic family and always assumed she would marry and have children. She received several marriage proposals when she was in her twenties, but she did not feel the men were right for her. After college she went to work for the Department of Health and Human Services. At the age of forty-seven she resigned from a management position to pursue her dream of becoming a lawyer; she now practices law.

"I became a career person pretty much through accident. What I thought I was going to do didn't happen. When I was thirty I thought, 'Ten years from now I'll be home taking care of kids.' I think it was about age thirty-five it began to hit me, 'Hey, you know, this may not happen. Maybe I'm not going to get married; maybe I'm not going to have a family.' From thirty-five on, as I neared my cutoff point of forty, I was most conscious of it. I'd think, 'Only three more years; only two more years.' I had my tubes tied when I was forty, because I knew if I *did* marry later, I'd try to get pregnant, even though the risks would be high for both me and the baby. I knew if there was a chance to have a baby, my emotions would override my judgment.

"I never envisioned myself as a single mother. My concept of having children has always been within the context of a family. I don't see myself being happy raising a child on my own, because part of the joy of having a child is sharing it with someone whose child it is, someone to whom that child is also dear. My concept is of a totality, a good marriage and children. To me it would be artificial to have a child as a single woman.

"Having never married, I never got to that point where having children was within reach and I couldn't have it. So it's a softer disappointment. Maybe that's the way to describe it."

Iris typifies many single childless women. Even though she wanted to be a wife and mother, she has made the most of her life. She is resourceful, independent, good-humored, and basically satisfied with her life. Few people who know her today could guess the disappointment she feels because she is childless.

"I Guess I'll Pass"

JACKIE'S STORY

Jackie, a bright, attractive thirty-eight-year-old single woman, is a physician who teaches in a southern California medical school. An only child, she was close to her father and frightened of her mother, a rigid, hostile woman, who resented Jackie's intelligence and beauty and constantly ridiculed her in front of friends and other family members. Because of the traumatic relationship she had with her mother, Jackie had no interest in mothering until she reached her midthirties. At that point she felt confident she would *not* pass on the family pathology if she mothered, and she finally felt she had something special to give to a child. Jackie talks with refreshing candor about modern women's deliberate choice whether to marry (which would give them the chance to have children) when the man is not *the* right man.

"At thirty-three I was involved with someone, and I thought we could have maybe five years together max. If I found someone like that today I might go ahead and have children. Five years, two kids, a decent person to share custody with. These days that might be okay, whereas at thirty-three it definitely was not.

"Some women do just decide, 'I will pick the best partner who comes because I want a family.' Several people have told me they decided this was the year they were getting married. If they set a deadline for December 31, the man may not be the most compatible person they dated, but he was there with the right inclination. Maybe they're just more reasonable than I am.

"One guy I went out with recently really wants a second family because he thinks he can get it right this time. On paper somebody might have paired us up on a blind date, but it didn't feel special to me. I said to myself, 'Suppose this is *your* shot at a family? Suppose this guy is the best parent-partner that you're going to find?' But I decided, 'If that's it, I guess I'll pass.'

"Sometimes I wonder if I think about it all too much. Maybe I should have just gone ahead and married and had a baby, even if I had doubts that the marriage would last. Maybe I should have just taken my chances.

"Right now I don't feel an urgency about the issue, but I can't say how I'll feel in a few years when I'm running out of time. I've thought about adopting. If I don't marry, that's probably what I'll do, because I do want to have a child."

Although Jackie begins by saying that now, at thirty-eight, she might compromise on marriage in a way she was not willing to do at thirty-three, when she talks about her most recent potential parent-partner she still decides to pass. Even though she knows her childbearing years are numbered, she will not marry unless the man is right for her. Other women, like Jackie, expressed their determination *not* to pass along family pathology. Jackie shows that it can be done. After years of therapy, she is now ready to be a nurturing, positive influence in a child's life.

"Going Through It Alone"

ERICA'S STORY

Erica is a forty-five-year-old single woman who *did* try to have her own child. She too grew up in a troubled family and has also worked hard, through therapy and other means, to undo the psychological damage caused by a father who abused her physically and sexually. She is a psychiatric social worker who works in a residential treatment program for disturbed adolescents. Erica loves her work, has many good friends, and travels a great deal. Even so, she judges herself (harshly, I think) because she is single.

"I feel I'm not normal because I haven't been able to get married. That's where it gets me. I haven't been able to do something that is healthy to do, to marry someone and say I do and I will. I haven't been able to go through that passage. And that's just devastating to me. As to not having a child, there's this part of me that I haven't been able to actualize, but I'm not less of a human being or a woman.

"I had decided if I wasn't married by the time I was thirty-seven, I would have a child on my own. I went to a doctor who does insemination, and the first time I got inseminated I got pregnant. Six weeks later I had a miscarriage. Going through the whole insemination process alone and then having a miscarriage was very hard, very traumatic. I got pregnant right away with the second insemination. And I carried the child longer, maybe two and a half months, and had another miscarriage. It took me a year to get through it to do it again. The third time I got pregnant right away, and three months later I had a sonogram and the doctor said, 'Well, it looks like clear sailing. This is the heartbeat, see it there. This looks fine.' That night I had a miscarriage, and it was just heartbreaking. A killer. My friends were supportive, but it's not like having a husband. Basically I was going through it alone.

"I didn't have the heart to try insemination again. I want to adopt a child, but somehow I'm afraid to do it without a partner. If I had a husband I'd definitely adopt. Then if the child had some kind of problem, hyperactivity or a medical condition, there'd be two of us to deal with it. But to chance it alone. It's scary."

Erica made initial inquiries about adopting, but then found herself immobilized, unable to take the next step. When I think of all she has been through, I am not surprised that she is reluctant to open herself to the possibility of more disappointment, more pain. She has already risked a lot to have a baby—three inseminations and three miscarriages—without success, and she did it alone.

INFERTILE WOMEN

Married infertile women are the women most frequently thought of when people think of childless women. Their ordeal is a prolonged one, often extending over many years. When pregnancy has not occurred after one year of intercourse, doctors usually recommend that the woman take her temperature every morning before rising and chart it on a basal temperature chart. Intercourse is then timed to coincide with ovulation. When conception still fails to occur, both the woman and her partner are subjected to a variety of diagnostic tests and procedures, some painful and unpleasant, others unlikely and amusing.

In the beginning they may laugh together when the man is told to ejaculate into a paper cup at the lab's restroom or when they have intercourse early on Monday morning (setting the alarm the night before) so the woman can hurry to her gynecologist immediately afterward for an exam. But as their sexual life is subjugated more and more to the demands of infertility studies and the attempt to conceive, humor may be replaced with frustration and discord. If the woman becomes obsessive about getting pregnant, her partner may feel her only interest in him (and in having sex with him) is to get pregnant.

If the woman is the one with the infertility problem, she may view herself as defective, unworthy, unlovable. She may worry that her husband will want a divorce so he can marry a woman who *can* have children. If her husband has the problem, she may feel angry and resentful toward him, even though she knows rationally that he is not deliberately keeping her from having a child. She may think of divorce herself or secretly entertain the idea of having an affair.

Even if the stress of infertility does not spill over into the relationship, the infertile woman experiences years of emotional highs and lows, as hopes rise with each new treatment and then fall with the onset of each menstrual cycle. As the months and years go by, such women often become frantic about having a baby. In their desperation to conceive, rational, educated women find themselves willing to try unlikely solutions. One woman confided she stood on her head after intercourse because a friend at work swore that was what finally worked for her.

Many women get depressed. They eat too much or lose interest in food; they sleep too much or dread sleep because they dream, distressingly, of babies; they lose interest in work and social activities. Especially during holidays, they avoid family gatherings where children, *other people's children,* will be present.

If you are an infertile woman, you know only too well the years of heartache and stress women endure in the futile hope that if only they try one more procedure, one more cycle of medicine, they *will* have a baby. Then, finally, they know that none of the new high-powered technology, none of the potent new drugs, will help *them.* Finally, they face the unacceptable fact that they will never conceive and give birth to a baby.

Some women then decide to try adoption. Others, who are already traumatized by the attempt to have children, decide they cannot, they will not, subject themselves to more years of uncertainty, more years of raised hopes and painful disappointment.

"Never Pregnant Once"

MARTI'S STORY

Marti is a forty-eight-year-old newspaper reporter who lives near Denver. She grew up in what she describes as a normal American family. Her father, a schoolteacher, and her mother, a homemaker, had two children, a boy and a girl. The family members have always enjoyed each other's company and still do. Her marriage is a second one for both her and her husband. She loves animals and owns five dogs of assorted sizes and shapes, two cats, and a goat. Although she was forty when she married her husband, she never doubted that she would get pregnant. She read and collected every magazine and newspaper article she could find about women over forty who got pregnant and had healthy babies.

"I suppose I went through a typical, unsuccessful infertility workup and treatment. I hardly remember all the different things we tried, the tests and the medicines and the surgical procedures. It just went on and on. Some procedures were really painful, though, and I started to wonder as the years went by, 'What am I doing to myself?' By the end I felt I was beating my head against a brick wall.

"The worst part was when I thought I was pregnant. I'd be late with my period, and I'd be so excited. I just *knew* this was it. When I'd call the lab to get the pregnancy test results, I'd get so choked up when it was negative that I could hardly talk. Never, not once, was I pregnant. Can you imagine? Never pregnant once!

"Sometimes in bed at night I'd sob and sob. My husband tried to comfort me, but I was inconsolable. And the dreams. Night after night, dreams about babies. It was awful. I'd wake up depressed and stay that way all day. I couldn't shake it.

"And then finally I had had enough. I couldn't stand any more. There might have been other things to try, but by then I'd given up. I knew I'd never have a baby.

"I get tremendous pleasure from having lots of animals. My mothering energy goes toward my pets, and they return it tenfold. My brother and his wife have three children, and I love being an aunt, but I still hurt about not being a mother. Just the other day I heard about a woman who is expecting her first child at forty-one, and I thought, irrational as it sounds, 'What does she know that I didn't know? What did she do that I didn't do?' It's as though everyone else knows some kind of secret, but no one will tell me what it is. Silly, isn't it?"

Marti finally decided, as do many other women, not only those with infertility problems, that she had to close the door on the possibility of having children. This assertion of will, taking control and ending a painful, unsuccessful process, often marks the beginning of resolution.

Adolescent Infertility

When a young woman learns as an adolescent that she is infertile because of congenital problems, the ramifications can be even more devastating than they are for adult women. Adolescence is the time when identity, especially sexual identity, is established. At its best the process is often difficult and is characterized by self-doubts and anxiety regarding one's desirability to and relationships with the opposite sex. When a young woman learns at this impressionable age that she has a physical abnormality that is intrinsically related to her sexual organs, she may have no way to deal with the information psychologically. Whether or not she suffers enduring emotional trauma will depend to a large extent on whether or not she has adults present in her life who can help her find meaning in her differentness.

Unfortunately, parents and other adults close to the girl are often overwhelmed by their own feelings. They cope by not talking about "it," hoping to lessen the trauma for her. Just the opposite happens. The girl may conclude from the adults' silence that the subject is taboo, too terrible to talk about, and so she refrains from sharing her feelings and concerns.

Teenagers are painfully self-conscious. Looking like, acting like, and feeling like one's peers permeates much of adolescent development, and the process is far more difficult for a teenager who *is different*. When a young woman learns she is infertile, does she share this information with her friends? If so, how will they view her? How and when does she tell boyfriends, or does she avoid boys altogether? Sharing with peers may ease her burden, but it also leaves her more vulnerable. The infertile adolescent girl will look toward her adult future in a different way than do other girls her age. If she had hoped to embrace the standard wife/mother role, she already has one strike against her. She knows that she cannot take motherhood for granted.

"A Deeply Flawed Person"

ELIZABETH'S STORY

Elizabeth is a thirty-five-year-old woman who teaches French at a small private college in Wisconsin. She is single and recently broke up with a man with whom she lived for five years. Elizabeth was an only child, and she describes her childhood as happy in most ways, her adolescence as turbulent. At age sixteen Elizabeth learned that she had a congenital defect that rendered her ovaries atrophic and nonfunctioning. Exploratory surgery revealed the abnormality after three years of medical investigations as to why her menstrual cycles stopped.

"My infertility has had a deep influence on my life. I still don't know all the ways it affected me. My menstrual cycles came to an abrupt halt when I was only fourteen, and it was a long, drawn-out process to determine what was wrong. I was young and didn't really know how to handle it. It was quite painful sometimes. The doctors were good people, but at times the hospital experiences, particularly when large groups of medical students peered at me as if I were a laboratory rat, were humiliating.

"Here is the sum total of the conversation in the doctor's office after the surgery when he had just explained what they found:

> MOM: You understand the implications of what Dr. Hager is saying, don't you?
>
> ME: Yes.

"We never spoke of it again until two or three years ago, and then only briefly. I can only guess at my parents' feelings about the whole thing.

"It came at a very vulnerable time in my sexual development. I had (and still in irrational moments do have) weird thoughts about my sexual identity and gender. I remember dealing with this by joking. My close high school friends who knew what I'd been through knew also that I was taking hormones. I think *I* am the one who made jokes about turning into a gorilla if I didn't take them, and other stuff like that. I never dealt with the pain that was there. There didn't seem to be any forum for dealing with it.

"I don't think it was loss that I experienced then. I was too young. It was confusion and humiliation and aloneness, feelings that I swallowed and tried to cover up with a cheerful attitude, but that didn't get me very far. I felt angry and confused and argumentative about all sorts of things during those years, but I never connected it to what was happening to me physically, and neither did my parents.

"The hardest part then and now was that I felt like I was not whole. I felt as though I was a deeply flawed person, that I couldn't hold my own in the world. This didn't arise from a feeling that women are supposed to have babies to be whole, though there is a *little* of that. I think it was simply that my body didn't *work,* and that there was no way for me to understand why it had happened to me."

Although Elizabeth's family was a normal, loving one, sixteen years passed with no discussion at all about her medical problems. If Elizabeth's feeling of not being whole had been directed only to her body, the damage to her self-esteem would have been limited, but she judged more than her body. She judged her entire being and found herself lacking. Fortunately, Elizabeth did find ways as an adult to move beyond her pain, and we hear from her again in Step 10.

Problem Pregnancies

Some of you had no trouble getting pregnant. You thrilled to the news of your pregnancy. You experienced the body changes pregnancy brings. You may even have felt your baby stir within you. But then problems arose during pregnancy or childbirth, and all your hopes evaporated; your joy changed to sorrow. In this section we talk about three kinds of problem pregnancies: multiple miscarriages, ectopic pregnancies, and stillbirths.

Women who experience problem pregnancies often tend to view their bodies as defective; they may even wonder if they have missing parts. It is understandable why they feel this way, because, in fact, their reproductive organs are *not* functioning in a normal, healthy way. But that does not equate with defective! The human body is an incredibly complex organism, not a manufactured product that can be recalled and replaced if it is defective. If you are childless because of problem pregnancies, be gentle with yourself. You are not less of a woman physically or less of a human being because of that. The inability to carry a pregnancy to term is heartbreak enough; do not punish yourself too. In Part III, "Ten Steps to Resolution," we talk about ways to stop self-blame.

Miscarriages

Many pregnancies end in miscarriages. Experts estimate that one out of every six terminates in the first trimester. Sometimes the woman is not even aware she is pregnant. Because miscarriages are so common and because many women experience normal pregnancies and childbirth after one or more, a miscarriage may be only a temporary setback rather than a harbinger of permanent problems. But not always. Sometimes one miscarriage is followed by another and another.

If you had a miscarriage, you may know that they are often painful. You may have experienced severe cramping, bleeding, and nausea over several days. If tissue remained in your uterus after the miscarriage, a surgical procedure known as a D & C (dilatation and curettage) of the uterus may have been required. But the physical pain of a miscarriage is often secondary to the emotional pain.

When a woman wants a baby, pregnancy is a time of joy, excitement, anticipation. The sudden loss of the baby brings disappointment and sorrow. Many years after a miscarriage, women—even those who have gone on to have children—remember the babies they lost. When pregnancy after pregnancy ends this way, the loss is even greater.

Even though a woman has had multiple miscarriages, when she learns she is pregnant again it seems impossible for her *not* to feel excited and hopeful. She may deliberately caution herself against these feelings, she may employ every psychological trick in her armamentarium to protect herself from the emotional pain of yet another lost pregnancy, but to no avail. Cliche though it is, hope *does* spring eternal. Even though she tries to contain her excitement when she learns she is pregnant, all her hopes, all her dreams about motherhood, all her longing for a baby revive of their own will.

Impossible as it seems *not* to hope, so, against all rationality, does it seem impossible not to blame oneself when a miscarriage occurs. Blame takes the form of wondering or saying to yourself, "Maybe I lost the baby because I———," or, "If only I hadn't———." If you have blamed yourself this way, you know that the self-accusations that fill the blanks are limited in number and scope only by your imagination. Other people in your life may intentionally or unwittingly feed this self-blame when they share their thoughts about why you miscarried. Ironically, the absurd reasons others offer as explanations may mirror the unreasonableness of your own accusations and eventually help you end the self-blame. One woman finally stopped punishing herself for supposed shortcomings when a friend told her she had lost two babies because she had not married the babies' father. She knew *that* explanation was ridiculous, which helped her realize her own self-blame was equally unfounded.

"Maybe If I Hadn't"

JEANNE'S STORY

Jeanne, who is thirty-six, was the oldest of four children. Because her father had trouble holding a job, her family had little money, even for essentials. When her mother worked two jobs, Jeanne was in charge of her younger brothers and sisters, and she tried to be a mother to them. She never resented taking care of them, even as an adolescent, and she always knew she wanted to be a mother. When she became pregnant as a senior in high school, she let her parents persuade her to have an abortion—a decision that she has regretted ever since. She married the first time when she was twenty-three and divorced three years later. She has been happily married to Jeff, her present husband, for seven years.

"I was so happy the first time I got pregnant, even though the baby's father didn't want to get married. I knew I could raise the baby by myself and give it a good home, but my parents thought I was too young. They wanted me to have an abortion, and because I loved them and didn't want to make them unhappy I did. I believed them when they said I'd have other babies later.

"In my first marriage I got pregnant twice and miscarried both times. I was heartbroken, but the marriage wasn't terrific, and after the divorce, when I met Jeff, I thought maybe it was for the best after all.

"Jeff wanted kids as much as I did. The first time we got pregnant we were so excited. I just knew that because Jeff and I loved each other so much and wanted a baby so badly, everything would go okay, but it didn't. I miscarried again. I guess I'm not a very fast learner, because when I got pregnant again I was just as excited. And just as heartbroken when I lost the baby.

"The next time I got pregnant I was determined to do everything right. I kept thinking, 'Maybe if I hadn't had sex, maybe if I hadn't drunk a glass of wine now and then, maybe if—' You accuse yourself. When I was pregnant and trying to keep the baby, I decided I needed to think all the right things. You know, not worry at all because if you have anxiety in your body you might miscarry. When I lost that baby I blamed myself because I hadn't thought pure enough thoughts. I know it's stupid—other women are stressed to the max and they have perfectly healthy babies—but I felt it had to be my fault.

"I blame myself most about the abortion, even though I believe women have the right to an abortion. But deep down I feel like God is punishing me because I killed my first baby. And I don't even really believe in God. It makes no sense, but that's how I feel.

"The last time I got pregnant I decided that if I lost this baby I would have a tubal ligation. I just couldn't take any more pain. I've had six pregnancies, and I have no babies."

Jeanne's emotional scars are still visible. She was either crying or trying to fight back her tears during our long talk together. She knows she needs counseling but has never been able to afford it. She feels very strongly that we need national health care, that no woman should have an abortion or a miscarriage or a tubal ligation without counseling.

Ectopic Pregnancies

Ectopic pregnancies, pregnancies in which the egg implants in the fallopian tube instead of the uterus, are much less common than miscarriages, but when they do occur they are life-threatening. Often neither the woman nor her physician knows she has a tubal pregnancy until she experiences acute abdominal pain. If an undiagnosed tubal pregnancy ruptures, massive internal hemorrhaging occurs, and the woman must be rushed to the emergency room, where, if she is lucky, she survives. Given the initial life-and-death crisis and the lengthy subsequent recovery, the woman initially may be thankful simply to be alive. It is later that she reacts to the lost pregnancy.

If you have experienced a ruptured ectopic pregnancy, you know how frightening and serious they can be. Your reproductive organs may have been badly damaged, and you may face partial or total loss of reproductive capacity. Even if you are able to get pregnant again, you may be understandably frightened that the same thing will happen again. You (and your husband and family) may decide that your life is not worth the risk of another pregnancy.

"So Many Missing Parts"

ISABEL'S STORY

Isabel is a forty-year-old physical therapist. She grew up in San Antonio, where she still lives, as do her parents and three brothers. She is an avid reader of romance novels, and she loves singing in the church choir. She has been married and divorced twice, and she currently lives alone.

"Believe it or not, I had two ectopic pregnancies, both during my first marriage. After the first one I thought, 'This can't happen again,' but it did. The second time it got stuck where the fallopian tube meets the wall of the uterus, which is fatal for the tube. It ruptured just really, really fast. By the time I got to the emergency room I had no pulse and no blood pressure because I was hemorrhaging so badly. I consider myself pretty lucky to be alive today.

"I have no tubes, one ovary, and most of a uterus left, so it would take extraordinary measures for me to get pregnant. I don't think it's going to happen. It really didn't bother me at the time I lost my fertility, because I was so sick. It's been mainly since my last divorce that I realize how much it does bother me that I can't have children. I always took it for granted that I'd be a mother.

"At times in my life I have been really hard on myself for being chopped up. After my first divorce, when I started dating again, I told men right away if it looked like we might get serious, because I didn't want to get involved with a man who wanted children and then suddenly I tell him I can't have kids. It wouldn't be fair. I guess it was a way to test them, too, to see if they wanted me even though I had so many missing parts.

"My second husband couldn't have children either because he had a problem with his sperm. In his first marriage they tried to have kids, and it was a real emotional issue for him that he couldn't. So that was kind of neat for both of us because we both had problems. We talked about adopting kids, but we divorced before we got around to it. I still want children, but I can't afford to adopt, so I don't think that's going to happen. My hope is that I'll marry some nice man who already has children, and I'll get to be the mother, or at least the stepmother, to his children. Now *that* might happen. I hope so. It's depressing to think I'll never have children."

Stillbirth

None of the women we have heard from so far has successfully carried a pregnancy to term or experienced childbirth, but any woman who has longed for a baby can imagine the sorrow of losing the baby after nine months of excitement, anticipation, and joy. Women who have stillborn babies experience a profound shock. They undergo the rigors of labor only to learn that there will be no baby to hold and love and nurture. When they leave the hospital, they must put away or give away the baby clothes they have ready; they must store or return the crib they chose so carefully. They must face the death of their baby. Even when I despaired about being childless, I knew I could, *would,* feel worse if I got pregnant and lost the baby, or if I had a child and something happened to that child.

"This Great Sense of Loss"

BEVERLY'S STORY

Beverly grew up in a small town in Kentucky. Her parents owned the only grocery store in town, and the family lived upstairs. While their parents minded the store below, Beverly and her twin sister played with their dolls and paper dolls for hours at a time. Beverly married her high school sweetheart and likes her life as a housewife. She is now forty-five.

"I always said I was going to have ten kids when I grew up. Both my sister and I wanted to have lots and lots of kids. My husband was never as big on kids as I was, but he knew it was important to me.

"We got married when I was twenty, and I didn't get pregnant for a long time. I don't know why. We live in a small town, and we didn't see any special doctors about it. Finally, about eight years into our marriage, I got pregnant, but I miscarried. I was heartsick. Then about four years later I got pregnant again. This time my doctor suggested we go to the city for an amniocentesis, which we did. When I found out I was going to have a son, I was ecstatic. I chose his name, Richard Lee, bought lots of little clothes for him, had his room all ready.

"Everything seemed normal during the pregnancy, and when labor started I went to the hospital. But the baby was stillborn. I was devastated. The nurses put me in a room away from the mothers with new babies. Then they brought my dead baby to me and asked if I'd like to hold it, and I said, 'No.' I wish someone had helped me at the time, helped me deal with my feelings and helped me hold my son. Maybe it would have helped me over this great sense of loss. The guilt I feel from thinking, 'I didn't want to hold my own baby,' hasn't passed. I can't even talk to my husband about it. You're the only person I've told.

"I still wish I had children, but I didn't try again. I couldn't go through that another time. I'm envious of my sister and my sisters-in-law who have children. Every time I attend a baseball game or a graduation or a wedding, I wonder how I would feel if it were my own child I was watching. I've never gotten over losing my son. It's an empty feeling."

When I picture Beverly alone in the hospital room, I want to be able to turn back the clock, be with her when they bring her her little son. I want to help her say good-bye. Like Elizabeth's parents, medical personnel are often overwhelmed by their own feelings of sadness when tragedy strikes and therefore are unable to help when help is needed most. Unfortunately, as we will see time and again, when sorrow and pain about losing, or not having, a baby go unresolved, the feelings linger and permeate a woman's life for years to come.

DISABILITIES, GENETIC PROBLEMS, AND ILLNESSES

Physical Disabilities

While it is true that many physically impaired women, including those with severe disabilities such as paraplegia, *do* become mothers, many others do not. Some disabled women are physically incapable of pregnancy and childbirth. Others are physically able to have children, but they cannot physically care for the children: they cannot hold or feed or pick up a child. Unless these women have the extensive financial resources necessary to pay someone else to provide such care, being a mother is a practical impossibility. Whatever the nature of the physical limitation, being childless is one loss superimposed on many other losses women with physical disabilities experience.

Such women may endure physical discomfort and poor health. They may depend on others, either family members or paid attendants, for help with daily living tasks. Physical movement and mobility are often restricted, which necessarily shrinks the physical world to which a disabled person has ready access. If you are a physically disabled woman, you know that daily activities other women take for granted—having a bath, mailing a letter, going to a movie—may require planning and/or help from others before you can undertake them.

Social relationships may suffer too. If an individual looks noticeably different, she may have to contend with stares and whispered comments from strangers. Some people feel uncomfortable when they are around people who are visibly different and try to avoid them. If relationships with such people matter to her, the disabled woman must assume the burden of allaying others' anxieties.

Restricted physical movement and travel make it more difficult to sustain social relationships, so a woman who is disabled is more likely to find herself socially isolated.

Many able-bodied people ignore or try to deny the sexuality of physically disabled people, preferring to believe that they have different needs and desires. Before my interview with Beth, who is physically impaired, I casually mentioned to a bright, sensitive male friend that I would be interviewing a woman who had been disabled all her life. I was surprised by his surprise. "Oh, surely she wouldn't have wanted to be a mother, would she?" he asked.

"I Would Have Given Anything"

BETH'S STORY

Beth is a fifty-six-year-old woman who is confined to a wheelchair. She lives with her elderly parents in a small town in Iowa. With few exceptions, she has been homebound all her life. She is part of a large, close-knit, deeply religious family. Beth smiled wistfully as she told me of her wish to have children.

"I would have given anything if I could have had children. Like everyone else growing up, I hoped that I would marry one day and have children. I would have if I'd married, I'm sure. I'm perfectly normal in that way, but I guess my physical handicap kept me from meeting anyone who would want to marry me. I wanted about a dozen children. I had names picked out. My first choices were Mary Ann and Ann Marie for girls, John and David for boys.

"I haven't been bitter or jealous, because I just accepted the fact that I can't have children. I didn't cry about it, but it was somewhat depressing. Other people don't really understand. I think you have to go through these things before you realize the heartache that goes with it. In my religion we believe in an afterlife, and people in my church say, 'Well, you'll have them in the next life,' but I'd rather have had children here. I don't know what it's like over there.

"It makes me so mad when I read in the newspaper or see on television the women who neglect their children and abuse them. They don't deserve to have children. It doesn't seem fair that they get to have children and I don't. I would have been a good mother. I know I would have.

"I do have five nephews and eight nieces, and I rejoice in their accomplishments, just as I would have done with my own children. Nieces and nephews are wonderful and fine, but it's not quite the same as having a child of your own. When I get older, it will be an even greater loss not to have a child. I worry about what I'll do when I lose my parents. I won't have children to lean on.

"Every day I sit by the window and see all these little children pass on their way from school, and they're just so cute. I think there'll always be a little pain there to realize I can't be a mother. I would have given anything to have a child, even one."

Of all the visual impressions that stayed with me from the interviews I conducted, none was as enduring as the picture of Beth in her wheelchair by the window watching the children pass on their way to school.

Genetic Problems and Illnesses

Two groups of women, women who know that they or their partners are carriers of recessive genetic defects and women who have certain serious illnesses, face an onerous choice. They must decide: do I have a child, knowing the child may be born with a serious, if not fatal, medical condition? Do I have a child, knowing that pregnancy may endanger my life and possibly the life of the child? If you have had to answer these questions yourself, you know the anguish involved.

Sometimes, as is the case with Tay-Sachs disease and sickle-cell anemia, the genetic defects occur almost exclusively in certain racial groups: Tay-Sachs occurs among Jewish people, sickle-cell anemia among African-American people. At other times the hereditary disorders are familial rather than racial, as is the case with cystic fibrosis.

Many women who face this dilemma seek genetic counseling, which helps to identify the probability of problems arising. If the odds are strongly in their favor, they may decide to go ahead with pregnancy. Two diagnostic procedures, amniocentesis, in which a sample of amniotic fluid is analyzed, and chorionic villus sampling, in which a sample of tissue from the placenta is analyzed, allow the diagnosis of certain conditions during pregnancy. If a woman learns that her baby will have Down's syndrome, muscular dystrophy, spina bifida, or hemophilia, she can decide to terminate the pregnancy at that point. Other women, including some who have seen a sibling suffer and die from a hereditary illness, decide, either with or without genetic counseling, that they will not risk giving birth to a child who has to endure a painful, debilitating, if not incurable illness.

A different group of women remain childless because *they* have serious medical problems that make pregnancy inadvisable. Because of potential complications, some women who have heart or kidney disease, diabetes, tuberculosis, or other major illnesses may be advised to forego pregnancy. Pregnancy places an additional physical strain on the body of women with these conditions and can destabilize the body's delicate metabolic processes. If women with these problems do become pregnant, their health and the health of the baby may be endangered. Other women may not have been advised to forego pregnancy, but because of their illnesses, they do not feel well enough to undertake pregnancy, childbirth, and the raising of a child. They need all their strength and energy simply to care for themselves.

"I Lost Part of Me as Well"

JOANN'S STORY

JoAnn lost her mother when she was eight years old. Although she felt close to her father and her paternal grandparents, who came to live with them after her mother's death, she always longed to have a mother. She has three brothers and sisters, who are much older than she is. JoAnn lives in a small town in Colorado with her second husband, to whom she has been married for six years. At thirty-eight, she is a contented homemaker who delights in crafts, sewing, and refinishing furniture. JoAnn has diabetes.

"When I found out I was pregnant the first time, I really was happy, though it took a while before I started getting excited about whether the baby would be a girl or a boy or wondered what kind of mother I would be, what kind of father my husband would be.

"My first baby was a little girl. Born at seven months, she lived only three hours. I had severe pneumonia at the time, so I wasn't aware of all the problems she was born with. Six years later my son was born when I was seven months pregnant. That was the last pregnancy I went through. We named him Patrick. He weighed one pound at birth and lived for two and a half months hospitalized in a neonatal intensive care unit. I spent all of that time living at the hospital. At the end we had to make a decision. Should we keep him on life support indefinitely? Or the next time he had a setback, should we take him off the machines? We let him go.

"Losing both babies was definitely a loss. It's hard to describe how you feel. There's a lot of pain. Each time I lost a baby, I lost part of me as well. It was like leaving the hospital, yet never really checking out. Always leaving something behind and wanting to return to pick it up. After I lost the second baby I had my tubes tied.

"I don't really know how I got through it. Religion is important to me, and I guess it helped me reach inside myself for strength

I never knew I had. I think that losing two babies was a factor in why my first marriage broke up. It was just too much for us to handle. And I guess I lost heart in some ways. I never thought of adopting children, not even with my husband now. I think I had to close the door on having children."

When JoAnn wrote to me, my first thought was that she did not fit the study. I was seeking women who would never be mothers, and JoAnn had given birth to two children. But when I considered that neither of her babies made it home from the hospital, when I considered the many days and nights and years of her life without children, I understood that JoAnn is a childless woman like the rest of us.

RELATIONSHIP ISSUES

Men Who Do Not Want Children

The dream of finding the right man and having a family takes an ironic twist for women who find that man, only to discover that he does not want children. Although there are many reasons why a man does not want children, often it is because he already has children from a previous marriage and has no wish to start another family. It is not unusual for the man to have had or to be planning to have a vasectomy. As more and more people divorce and remarry, increasing numbers of women find themselves in this predicament.

If you are in love (or in the process of falling in love) with a man who does not want children, you are faced with a difficult choice: do you choose the man who *is* a part of your life and very much a reality, or do you end the relationship to pursue your dream of the ideal situation, namely, a loving husband *and* children. If you choose the latter, you must again seek a suitable mate who wants to have children, and while love at first sight and marriage soon after are possible, meeting the "right" man, falling in love, and deciding to marry could take years. Even then there is no guarantee that the couple will be able to have children. If the woman renounces the man she loves and does not find a more amenable replacement, she may live the rest of her life alone, without a partner and without a child.

The woman who decides to marry the man she loves may tell herself, and believe it to be true, either that she will persuade him to change his mind about having children later or that having a child does not really matter that much to her. Often she understands completely why the man does not want more children: he has been through a lot with the children he already has, or at his age (the man is usually older than the woman) he wants more freedom and less responsibility. This is a situation where women often take care of the men they love at their own expense. Unwittingly, they attend to the man's needs and wishes before they attend to their own. They fail to see that their *own* needs and wishes are no less important, no less crucial to the well-being of the relationship.

The woman (and her man) may be surprised when the issue of having children emerges as a highly charged one that threatens either the woman's peace of mind and happiness and/or the relationship. This may happen suddenly or over a period of years, as the intense longing for a child replaces the bloom of romance and a new marriage. Often the woman then blames her husband for depriving her of the child she wants.

"What Have I Done?"

GWEN'S STORY

Gwen *did not* always assume she would be a mother. Her father left her mother for another woman when Gwen was four, and her mother struggled to raise three children alone. Gwen accepted her mother's admonitions to get an education, have a career, and never depend on a man. It was not until she neared thirty that Gwen began to think she would also like to have a child. When she met her husband, Don, who is eleven years older than Gwen, they developed an immediate and powerful connection. Her husband had two adolescent children from a previous marriage and did not want more children. This is Gwen's first marriage. She is thirty-five and works in New York City as an account executive for a large insurance brokerage firm, a position she loves.

"When Don and I first discussed the possibility of buying a place and living together, he expressed concern that I would want children, and he knew he did not. I could completely understand why he felt that way. I thought, 'My God, if I had two teenage kids, and they were going through what his are going through, I wouldn't want to start again.'

"At that time I didn't feel an immediate, pressing need to have a child. We discussed the subject infrequently, perhaps three times, over the next year and always returned to the same stalemate. I felt more certain that I wanted to be with Don than I did about the possibility of future children.

"We bought a place, and shortly after we moved in Don had a vasectomy. Although we had discussed it, when it happened I remember feeling shocked and numb. I thought, 'What have I done?!' Suddenly the reality of it sank in. I felt this tremendous sense of loss and loss of power over my own destiny. I'd given up something and didn't know I had given it up until it was too late.

"I was very angry at Don. Even now when the topic comes up, which it does occasionally, I can still get really angry about it. I still resent it, and him, on some level. And the immediacy and force of my anger remind me that the decision may not be final for me. I still feel more strongly that I want to be with him, but I also know that there's the possibility that the balance could shift.

"If I had known at that time what I know now, or even what I felt the day after Don's vasectomy, I would have fought to prolong the decision making. I didn't make the decision lightly, but it amazes me now that I was willing to make it without pushing for more conversation about it. Don and I have discussed all these issues in circles, and he insists that if *he* had known, he wouldn't have pushed for such a final decision at that time. His memory is clearly different than mine, which I find very common in the annals of men and women.

"It was too easy for me to put myself in his place rather than putting myself in my place. That's the big mistake I made, I think now, looking back. I was looking at it too logically. I put my needs aside for the relationship."

Gwen's anger relates primarily to the loss of power over her own destiny. She concedes the possibility that she might have opted not to have children. If *she* had made the decision, not had it thrust on her, her feelings about being childless would be very different. This theme surfaced with many women, not only those with partners who did not want children. Feeling powerless made the adjustment to childlessness much more difficult. Gwen is a fair person and knows, rationally, that she is not sticking to an agreement she made of her own free will. Her situation is a classic one where the heart overrules the mind.

Men Who Have Behavioral Problems

Some women remain childless because all their romantic liaisons are with men who have severe behavioral problems, men who are "totally unsuitable" fathers. Obviously there are many other women *with children* who are involved with the same kind of men. This latter group chose to have children whether or not the man in question was a prime candidate for fatherhood. But the women I talked to were unwilling, in spite of their often intense desire to have children, to parent with men they believed would be inadequate fathers.

If you are involved with a man who is habitually unfaithful, drunk, on drugs, broke because he gambles or is out of work, in jail, hiding so he does not go to jail, or violent, your life is probably in an uproar much of the time. That kind of tumultuous home life cannot provide the stability and security children need. It is not surprising that many women choose *not* to bring a child into such an environment.

What may surprise an objective observer is that women stay in such situations. Although the motivation for doing so varies for each woman, the underlying dynamic is the woman's unresolved emotional needs, which she tries to resolve through her repetitive behavior or through staying in the relationship. A woman who saw her alcoholic father destroy himself and his life may try, symbolically, to rescue him through involvement with alcoholic men whom she thinks she can help. A woman who was abused as a child does not believe that she is lovable or that she deserves love and happiness. If she *were* lovable, if she did deserve happiness, her parent(s) would not have abused her. So she involves herself in relationships with men who mistreat her, thus confirming that her own badness is the reason her parents treated her the way they did.

Although the women have problems in their relationships with men, often these problems do not spill over into other areas of their lives. They may be successful at their work, they may have satisfactory relationships with family and friends, and they may have the potential to be good mothers. The women I talked to believed, and I agreed with them, that they would have been good mothers. The fact that they chose *not* to bring a child into a home where love and security could not be taken for granted, where the adult's needs—not the child's—would be primary, shows that in this area they made unselfish, mature judgments.

Friends and family often criticize women in such relationships. These concerned others feel infuriated when they see the woman mistreated, worry that she is wasting her life, warn her that the future will be one ugly crisis after another. Sometimes women who involve themselves with problem men see their part in the pattern. They know they have chosen such men, they may understand the dynamics of why they make that choice, and yet they are still driven to perpetuate the pattern. If you see yourself in this picture, you know that understanding does not always lead to change. In this as in many areas of our lives, when behavior is motivated by unresolved emotional needs, the obvious is not always easily executed.

"Absurd Choices"

CHRISTIANA'S STORY

Christiana is a bright, attractive, thirty-four-year-old woman who has her own computer consulting firm in Houston. Christiana's mother, whom she describes as a brilliant, creative woman, struggled with a drinking problem and addictions to psychiatric drugs for nearly twenty years before her death. Christiana says she grew up "gravely impressed" by her mother's situation and felt in some way responsible for her mother's problems. Christiana divorced after a brief marriage when she was in her twenties. She had one miscarriage during that marriage.

"I've thought a lot about the reasons I don't have kids, and the main reason is that I was never able to form a lasting bond with a suitable father. Only recently I realized that my romantic preferences are closely tied to my experiences growing up in an alcoholic family. Often adult children of alcoholics end up either substance abusers themselves or enablers and caretakers of others who drink or take drugs. I'm a caretaker. It's really astounding to look back on my own romantic history and admit just how consistently I've chosen men who abused drugs and alcohol, or with similar family histories of highly dysfunctional behavioral problems such as extramarital affairs and gambling.

"Needless to say, these men had serious personal problems of their own to work out before they were ready for fatherhood. I'm glad that I cut my losses with all of them after two years or so, because *not one* has gone on to make healthy changes in these areas since we were together. As far as I know, they're all still drinking and taking drugs or cheating on their present girlfriends and wives. I couldn't see raising a child under those circumstances then, and I can't see it now.

"My latest love affair was also the most disastrous. To my credit, I realized early on that I'd made a mistake and tried to extricate myself quickly. Unfortunately, this guy was really tenacious. He threatened suicide, he was physically violent, and he stole money from me and my father to support a drug habit that at the time I didn't even know he had.

"One of the tricks he pulled to keep me tied to him was trying to get me pregnant by intentionally sabotaging birth control during a time when I was fertile. He knew that due to my strong feelings about abortion I would probably go through with the pregnancy. Anyway, he put a condom on in such a way that he knew it would be pulled off easily during intercourse. I freaked out when I saw the results. Without telling him, I went to my gynecologist for the morning-after pill.

"There are times when I feel tremendous sadness at never having found the right partner with whom to raise a family. I also feel some shame at having made such absurd choices, but I've been dealing with that issue very directly in terms of seeing my dysfunction and realizing that I don't need to keep making the choices that put me in a no-win situation."

Christiana has not entirely given up hope of having a child, but she thinks it is unlikely, since she has no suitable parent-partner in her life right now. She is close to her father, who tolerates but cannot understand her choice of men. We will hear from Christiana again in Step 5, "Talking to Significant Others."

LESBIAN WOMEN

Many lesbian women want children, but few have them. They may be childless for the same reasons that heterosexual women are childless—infertility problems, illnesses or disabilities, partners who do not want children—but in addition they face complex issues unique to their situation.

The single most important issue lesbian women consider when they think of having children is the potential effect on a child of growing up in a homophobic society. Homophobia, which manifests itself as a critical, often hostile, attitude toward gay people, pervades much of society. Lesbians who want children may be unable to find nonjudgmental child care. When their children go to school, there may be no other children who are also identified as children of lesbians. As the children grow up, they may be stigmatized and ostracized because of their nontraditional family. They may even be physically endangered, a victim of the unprovoked attacks to which gay people are often subjected. Closer to home, the parents and siblings of lesbians may not support the decision to have a child. They may be ashamed to have a pregnant lesbian daughter or sister; they may not accept the child.

A second major consideration, especially for couples who have a committed relationship, is the question of the role of the woman who is not the biological mother. Will there be competition for the all-important role of mother? How will the coparent define her position to people outside the relationship? How will she answer the question, "Are you the baby's mother?" Will she feel like a minor figure in the child's life? Will others see her that way? Can she proudly announce and share her excitement about the pregnancy with her coworkers? During the pregnancy, will she be welcomed as the coparent at the doctor's office and in the delivery room?

Legal rights are another ambiguous area. Although the nonbiological parent may be emotionally involved in raising the child, may assume financial responsibility and share equally in child care, under the law this parent may have no rights. Women who live in states that allow gay people to adopt children can protect their rights through adoption, but not all women have such recourse available to them.

The question of the sperm donor must also be addressed. In some parts of the country, lesbians are welcome at clinics that offer insemination, but not all women have access to these clinics. Of course, male donors may also be found informally. Many lesbians want the child to be a biological product of both partners. To ensure this, one woman will have a brother or other male relative donate sperm that will be used to inseminate the other woman. Friends, sometimes gay men, may also donate sperm.

It takes many lesbian women and couples years before they can deal with society's condemnation of their sexual orientation and the internalized self-blame and guilt that result. By the time they come out of the closet, they are often in their late thirties, which means the biological time clock is ticking away.

Because of the many difficulties they would have to face if they had children, most lesbians, like most single women, keep the issue at arm's length. By *not* allowing free reign to the dream of having a child, they protect themselves from heartache and disappointment.

"That Desire Is There"

SUE ELLEN'S STORY

Sue Ellen is a twenty-six-year-old waitress who lives in the rural South. She grew up on a farm, where her parents and two younger siblings still live. She has two older married sisters and an older brother, who is also gay. She is close to everyone in her family, all of whom accept the fact that she and her brother are gay. During high school Sue Ellen dated boys and was sexually active with one boyfriend, but both the dating and sexual activity held no interest for her. She realized she was a lesbian when, at twenty-one, she fell in love with a woman she met at work.

"The question of having children has come up in several relationships I've been in. I think most lesbians *do* want to have children. That desire is there, even though most don't go ahead.

"The gay community almost everywhere is still struggling to find its own values. It's very rare to see a couple here that stays together for long. I think because marriage isn't legal for lesbians, there's not the total commitment. The back door is always open. So that's one consideration about having a baby. Your partner may not be there.

"Most people here are real conservative. A lot of my friends don't even tell their families that they're lesbians. Adopting a child would be real hard, if not impossible, in this area, and I don't have any information on artificial insemination.

"I was brought up with traditional values, and I've always felt I want one partner in my life for a long time. I'm in a new relationship that will probably be long term; we've been together four months now, and we're talking about having a minister do a union ceremony. I would want a child to be a product of both partners; I would want the child to show the love and connection between me and my partner. Since that's not possible, I guess my feeling is more not to have a child, even though I want one.

"My new partner was married before she realized she was gay, and she has two children. The children don't live with her, but I have contact with them. I won't be their parent, but I can take the role of a friend who looks to see what their needs are. I like that."

Sue Ellen is still a young woman and may yet decide to have a child if she does find the long-term relationship she desires. The question of having children tends to surface seriously with lesbians when a couple has been together for five or so years. As more and more lesbians *do* have children, society will have to accommodate these nontypical families—willingly or unwillingly—and Sue Ellen may find that even her conservative small town will change.

"I'm Not Ready to Let Go of the Dream"

TINA'S STORY

Tina, who is thirty-eight, is one of four children. Her father, an attorney, was the mayor in the Nebraska city where she grew up. Her mother is a social worker. Tina completed her education in the Midwest and moved to San Francisco ten years ago, because she wanted to be able to live openly as a lesbian. She met Gloria, her partner, soon after she arrived, and they have been together for nine years. Tina works as an attorney for the state of California.

"I mothered my younger brothers and sister a lot when I was growing up, so I didn't feel a real push to have my own child until I was close to thirty. Even then it was always going to happen down the road, after I reached a certain point in my career, but I knew I wanted a child sometime.

"I'm fortunate because my parents are very accepting of my being a lesbian, and they like and respect Gloria. Even so, when I've mentioned my wish to have a child, they say, 'Why would you want to do that to a child?' I know what they mean, because a child of a lesbian couple faces many potential problems. You have to think seriously about the social pressures on a child who grows up in a nontraditional family. San Francisco is a liberal community, but even so you have to wonder what it would be like for a child. I'd hate to have my child taunted and ostracized. It's hard enough for an adult to cope with being different. I know it's taken me a long time to accept who I am, and I think how difficult it would be for a child to have lesbian parents.

"If we do have a child, it's important to me that the child be a biological product of both of us. Even before I met Gloria, I came up with a plan. We would have my partner's egg extracted and fertilized by my brother's sperm, and then the fertilized egg would be implanted in me. That way we would both have biological ties to the child. My partner would be the biological mother, and I would be the birth mother.

"Lately, the last year or so, I've really started to appreciate what a good life Gloria and I have. We both love our careers and work hard at them; we come and go as we please. If we had a child, our life-styles would have to change, so I don't know what we'll decide. Although she doesn't say so, I sense that Gloria would rather not have a child, but I'm not ready to let go of the dream yet."

Tina's ambivalence about having a child came through clearly when we talked. She *does* want a child, but the factors she discussed weigh heavily on her mind. Since she and Gloria bought a house and got a dog, Tina's nurturing energy has had a focus, the dog, whom she adores. She is clear in her own mind that if she does not have a child, she will definitely quit the job she has now and find one that allows her to work more directly with people, perhaps legal aid. If she does not have a child, she must redirect her nurturing energy.

Biological Alarm Clock

The notion of a biological alarm clock ticking away has come to symbolize a woman's anxious awareness that her childbearing years are nearing an end, that she is running out of time. While women can and do have children into their late forties, doing so is the exception rather than the rule.

Physical complications that interfere with pregnancy are more prevalent in older women. (In the context of pregnancy, older means thirty-five to forty.) Twenty-year-olds trying to get pregnant usually succeed; forty-year-olds often do not. As women age, if they have not had children, they are more likely to develop endometriosis, a condition that frequently interferes with conception and pregnancy. Benign tumors of the uterus are not uncommon. Menopause is another factor that must be reckoned with. When women reach their forties, menopause may be waiting in the wings, and an early-onset menopause can affect ovulation, which in turn makes conception more difficult. Acutely aware of the inexorable, biological limits to childbearing, childless women hear the alarm clock ticking away.

Many women set a deadline for themselves, a given age after which they will not get pregnant because of the increased risk to themselves and to a baby. In the past, before "older" mothers became commonplace, many women considered thirty to be a cutoff point for having a first baby. Today forty or even forty-five is more likely. Interestingly, the sense of time running out is not necessarily age related. A physician who wrote felt she still had many years left. She said, "I feel like I lost some years in medical school because the social part of my life was on hold. I hear the numbers, and I know I'm thirty-eight. When I look in the mirror, I know I don't look like

I did at twenty-five. But even so I feel my calendar's starting now." Other women decide at thirty-eight that their time is up.

Some women postpone having children for career reasons or wait simply because their lives are satisfactory and they feel no pressing need to have children. As their twenties and thirties slip by, these women take little notice of the passing years (in relation to childbearing), believing that they will have children later, when they are ready. Often the sense of urgency strikes suddenly. It is now or never, they feel. Many women who postponed childbearing will get pregnant once they try; they will have the children they desire. Many others will not; they will face regret and remorse because they waited too long.

"Always Tomorrow"

ROBERTA'S STORY

Roberta grew up in Baltimore, the youngest child of a family who was often on welfare. She was determined to chart a different course for herself and at forty-six is now the principal of a primary school in Baton Rouge. She finds her work gratifying and knows she is proficient at it. She has been in a good marriage for seventeen years, has many friends, and is close to her family.

"I always thought that I wanted children, but it was always tomorrow. I had been pregnant when I was twenty and in college, but the relationship was very inappropriate for me, and he had no interest in marrying me. Abortions were illegal at that time, but he found a doctor in New Orleans and took me there. I got an infection and almost died.

"When I was twenty-nine, I met my husband, and we married several years later. He had four children from his first marriage, but he was up for having more. We decided to have a family, but I always said, 'Later,' and continued with my career. Our marriage went on, and I just kept putting it off and not thinking anything of it.

"When I was thirty-seven I said, 'Maybe this is the time,' and I went off of birth control. My friends had started having kids, and I decided it was about time for me to do it. We tried for two years to get me pregnant and couldn't. I had all the tests done. My tubes weren't blocked; his semen was fine. I was one of those cases where there was no known reason why I didn't get pregnant. We kept trying, but now I've started into menopause, so it's not going to happen. I'm sorry I waited so long. I might have had problems when I was younger, but somehow I doubt it. Now I have to live with the feeling that I just frittered my childbearing years away. I'd tell other women who do what I did, 'You don't have as much time as you think.' "

Roberta, like many other career women, postponed childbearing because the present time never seemed right for starting a family. Unfortunately, many women now *do* have to choose, either to pursue a satisfying career *or* take time out for a family. I hope the day will come when society's attitudes and structures change, when everyone assumes that most women, like most men, will have both careers *and* families, when quality child care exists for everyone. In the meantime, if you *know* that you want to have children, and your life situation is such that you *can* have children, think twice about waiting. Women who want children and procrastinate until it is too late often regret the years they let slip by. The young believe they have all the time in the world. As we get older and wiser, we know otherwise.

PART THREE

Ten Steps to Resolution

STEP 1 *Acknowledging and Experiencing the Loss*

STEP 2 *Understanding the Loss*

STEP 3 *Surviving the Loss*

STEP 4 *Letting Go of Blame*

STEP 5 *Talking to Significant Others*

STEP 6 *Using Available Resources*

STEP 7 *Rechanneling Mothering Energy*

STEP 8 *Including Children in Your Life*

STEP 9 *Maximizing the Advantages of Childfree Living*

STEP 10 *Embracing the Quest for Feminine Wholeness*

Introduction to Resolution

THE GOALS OF RESOLUTION

The two primary goals of resolution are ending the pain of childlessness and moving beyond the loss, getting on with the business of living. Not all women experience pain, but those who do know how debilitating it can be. Women whose energies and emotions are bound up in the heartache and loss of being childless often put their lives on hold for years. Childlessness is a great loss, but it does not have to mean a lifetime of pain. The second and primary goal of resolution is even more crucial than the first. Going beyond the negative, going beyond the loss, creating a rich, full, satisfying life is the great challenge of resolution.

WHAT RESOLUTION IS AND IS NOT

Many people have mistaken notions about resolution.

Resolution does not mean you will be glad you are childless. On the contrary. Even women who resolve their feelings of loss continue to wish they had had children. That basic choice for how you wanted to live your life will not have changed. What will change is that it becomes a *past* issue, not a current one. Resolution is the difference between "I wanted a child" and "I want a child."

Resolution does not mean that you will have no feelings about being childless. You will not one day cross a line into an exalted place beyond the reach of human emotions, a higher emotional plane where you have no feelings about being childless.

People often ask me if it is really possible for women who wanted children to resolve their feelings to such a degree that they feel no pain about being childless. My answer is an emphatic "Yes!" When they ask if that means women have no feelings about being childless, my answer is very different. Often there is fleeting sadness, lingering wistfulness. The healing process here parallels the healing that takes place following a death.

When someone we love dies, we initially feel that we will never be completely happy again. The loss is so profound that we believe we will feel an emptiness for the rest of our lives. Then one day we realize that hours have gone by when we were not aware of the loss; later entire days pass without sorrow; eventually feelings of loss no longer permeate our lives. But sometimes, unexpectedly, there is fleeting sadness. We miss the loved one, long to talk to him or her. On occasion we may even cry. But the feeling passes. We never return to the sense of overwhelming loss.

And so it is with childlessness. You will find that the pain passes; you will find life well worth living. But there will be times of passing wistfulness. When you least expect it, you think of the child you wanted, and a shadow drifts across your life, like the shadow cast when a cloud drifts across the sun, but the shadow passes, and the sun shines again.

Resolution is not a destination but a journey. Often we think of journeys as being less important than destinations, but they are not. When we are young, many of us dream of meeting Prince Charming and living happily ever after. When we are in school, we focus on graduation and cannot wait until the big event. As we mature, after we meet Prince Charming, after we graduate, we come to realize that what really matters is not the meeting but the days that constitute happily ever after, not the graduation but the experiences of school days and the experiences that follow graduation. In other words, it is the striving, the daily living that gives meaning and shape to our lives, not just the achievement of a particular goal. Resolving your feelings about being childless means living the many days of your life as well as you can, as fully as you can; it means minimizing the losses of childlessness and maximizing the assets of your life.

Using the Steps

As you embark on the long, intricate, inward journey of resolution, remember that it has many highs and lows. At times you will see your way clearly; at other times you will lose your way. Do not get discouraged; do not give up.

Not all steps will have equal significance for you. If you never blamed yourself or others, Step 4 will have little to offer you. If you always turned to and had the support of close friends or family, just skim Step 5. If you know the joy of having children in your life, you may be surprised to learn that not all women do. When any step seems obvious to you, when it is something you have known or been doing all along, then chalk it up to your being on the right track. Trust yourself. You will know whether you are avoiding a step or if you do not really need it.

You should start at Step 1, proceed to Step 2, and so on, because there is a natural progression to the healing process. Timing for the different steps is all important. If you decide early on to jump to Step 7 or Step 9 without doing the grief work implicit in the first steps, your attempts to rechannel mothering energy or maximize the advantages of childfree living will be only rationalizations at a superficial level. They may even delay the healing process, because they help you deny your loss. A certain amount of grief work, of letting go, *must* take place first. Otherwise, the intention comes from the will and the mind, not from a resolved heart. I cannot overemphasize how important this initial grief work is; it is the foundation for the entire resolution process. In the proper time, all the steps do work, but not until you have dealt with underlying feelings.

You will not complete one step, finish with it forever, then move on to the next, finish with it, and so on. You will return to certain steps repeatedly, working them at a deeper level each time. For example, you do not complete Step 1 and never have to deal with feelings of loss again. You will deal with loss many times, but the intensity of the feelings and their power to wound will lessen each time.

You may resonate to the challenge of certain steps. You may discover in Step 2 that a primary dynamic for you in childlessness is attending to and nurturing your own inner child, who is deeply wounded, and that this need permeates all your life. Or you may realize in Step 7 that you not only need to redirect your mothering energy but also need to challenge and exploit your creative abilities in other significant parts of your life. You will know you need to rework certain steps if your energies and emotions keep returning to an issue you thought you had resolved once and for all.

These steps contain no magic; they offer no easy panacea. Each of us must find and follow her own path to resolution. But if you use the steps, they will guide you as you search for and find your path. They will help to light the way.

STEP ONE

Acknowledging and Experiencing the Loss

"I will never be a mother. I will never have a child."

I remember the day I said those words to myself for the first time. I cannot describe the sense of loss that filled my soul. Yet I knew I had to say the words, had to face my reality, one I had dreaded and fought against for more years than I cared to remember. If I had had the energy, there were more medical procedures, more extreme measures I could have tried, but I had decided where there was hope there was pain, and I had had enough of both.

When I said those words, "I will never have a child," I dealt the death knell to Jenny, the little girl who had lived in my heart for years. I clamped a tight lid on my sorrow, determined to get on with my life, and it was months before I allowed myself to mourn for what would never be:

- never to feel my baby stir within my body
- never to hold my newborn child
- never to feel her nursing at my breast

- never to caress her, stroke her cheek
- never to feed her strained squash or prunes or green beans
- never to buy yellow rubber ducks for her bath
- never to rock her to sleep, tuck her into bed
- never to choose wallpaper with zoo animals or clowns for her room
- never to see her take her first step
- never to read a favorite bedtime story over and over and over again
- never to hear her laugh, to hear her talk
- never to comfort her when she falls down or is ill
- never to hear her little voice saying, "I love you, Mommy," and feel her arms around my neck
- never to take her to a first day at school
- never to receive a picture she drew just for me on Mother's Day
- never to take her to the zoo, the beach, the playground
- never to take her anyplace
- never to hold her on my lap, safe within the circle of my arms
- never to watch her skip a rope, play softball, perform in a church or school play
- never to listen to her chatter on the telephone as a teenager
- never to have philosophical discussions with her when she discovers the world's imperfections

- never to see her go to her first formal dance
- never to see her graduate from high school or college
- never to see her marry or have her own children
- never to share with my grown-up daughter what I have learned about God and love and friendship and cooking
- never to . . .
- never to . . .
- never to . . .

A SIGNIFICANT LOSS

Women who wanted children experience loss that is deep and lasting, yet many childless women (and others) fail to acknowledge the true depth of the loss. The primary reason why the loss is minimized is because a childless woman's children never had a physical reality; they existed only in the woman's heart and mind. We all know the sorrow women feel if they lose a child because of an illness or an accident. We all know the sorrow women feel when a premature baby dies, when a baby is stillborn, when a woman miscarries. The loss childless women feel is another step on the continuum. To lose a child under any circumstances is to lose a loved one. When a childless woman loses the children she longed to have, it means she will never know the tender moments, the funny moments, the lifetime of shared experiences she would have had with her children. Nor will she have memories of these times together to comfort her in the absence of the loved one.

Childless women also lose the part of themselves that would have been a mother. Motherhood provides women the opportunity to explore who they are: their capacity for growth, their ability to love selflessly, their skill at guiding and influencing a child. Many of us hoped that as mothers the noblest, most honorable parts of our character would blossom and grow, that we would reach our highest level of functioning as mature human beings. When you consider the emotional investment you have made in your dream of being a mother, an investment that may well span decades of your life, you will understand why you cannot lightly turn and walk away from that part of yourself.

THE NEED TO MOURN

Just as the physical body must slowly heal after an accident or serious illness, so our hearts must slowly heal after a significant loss. I think of it as healing from the inside out. It is possible—some people are more skilled at it than others—to put on a good front after a significant loss. Doing so enables a grieving person to get through a day at work or go grocery shopping without exhibiting her sorrow to the world. The danger arises when we hide our feelings from ourselves. Emotional pain that is pushed below the surface and ignored will not go away. It extracts a toll in terms of energy, ability to form meaningful relationships, and a sense of well-being. It often resurfaces later.

Time and again in my clinical practice I have seen the long-term effects of problems that were either ignored or dismissed as unimportant when they first appeared. It may have been behavioral problems with a child—stealing, aggressiveness, withdrawal—or problems in a marriage—one partner with an explosive temper, a drinking problem, infidelity. By the time the problem is brought to therapy, individuals have endured years of heartache, patterns are entrenched, and bad feelings have intensified to such an extent that change is difficult if not impossible.

That is why it is crucial to mourn a loss when you first experience it. The only way to heal, heal from the inside out, is to allow yourself to feel the sadness, the fear, the disappointment. There is no other way.

In the book *Without Child: Experiencing and Resolving Infertility,* by Ellen Sarasohn Glazer and Susan Lewis Cooper, one woman, Teri Flinn, who has a child but has been unable to have the second child she desperately wants, talks of her plan to buy the cutest Cabbage Patch doll she can find, dress it in special baby clothes, kiss it good-bye, place it in a tiny box, and bury it. She will do this alone, say her good-byes alone, cry her tears alone. I understand her need to do this. When we lose someone we love, we feel a spiritual need to express our sorrow, to say good-bye. Even though our children never came to be, we did know and love them in our hearts, and we need to say good-bye.

THE TEMPTATION TO AVOID MOURNING

Because your feelings are so painful, you may be tempted to rush through this step or avoid it altogether. Do not do this! I cannot emphasize enough the importance of this first step; it is the foundation for all the steps that follow. However difficult it is, you need to let yourself mourn the child you never had, let yourself feel what you lose when you bury your dream of being a mother.

Do not expect it to be easy. You may cry a lot. You may feel great sadness and despair. For a period of time you may feel depressed. Or you may just feel flat, without energy or interest in your life. You may want to be alone. There is no right or wrong way to feel. Accept whatever feelings you have. Trust yourself that you have a reason for feeling the way you do. Also trust that you will not always feel the way you do now.

FEAR THAT THE FEELINGS WILL OVERWHELM US

Some women knowingly or unknowingly deny, minimize, or avoid their feelings of loss. They do so for several reasons. The first reason is because the feelings that accompany loss are not pleasant. No one likes to feel sad or depressed or flat; we would prefer to feel happy and upbeat. The second reason is that women fear being overwhelmed by the intensity of their feelings. They fear they will open a Pandora's box and be unable to get the lid back on. This is a realistic concern for some women. Just as it is important to feel your feelings, it is equally important not to let yourself drown in them. You need to find a balance. One woman I interviewed understood the dilemma well. She allowed herself one day a week to cry, mourn, feel sorry for herself, and indulge her feelings. The other six days she locked the door on sadness and got on with the rest of her life.

How you choose to acknowledge and experience your loss is an individual decision. If you experienced childlessness as traumatic, you may have constructed elaborate defenses to protect yourself from feeling the loss, and you may be frightened at the prospect of dismantling those defenses. Take it one step at a time. If you feel overwhelmed, pull back for awhile. You may need the support of another person: a family member, a close friend, a therapist, or a minister, priest, or rabbi.

Some of you may not be ready to take this first step. You may still have reason to hope that you will have a child (even though in your heart you doubt it), or you may feel you do not have the emotional strength and energy necessary to open your heart to the pain. Trust yourself if you feel this way. No one else can determine when and how you should proceed. Just remember that at some point you *will* need to acknowledge and experience your loss.

HOW TO GET IN TOUCH WITH YOUR FEELINGS

If you have denied your loss for a long time, you may have difficulty getting in touch with your feelings. Try writing your own list of "never to . . ." items. For one week, remember all your fantasies of being a mother, remember all the things you looked forward to doing with your child, and write them down.

Or try writing a letter to your child. Tell him or her about your wish for a baby, of the relationship you longed to have. A variation of this exercise is talking to your child. One woman's therapist had her imagine and talk to the child she wanted to have, a powerful experience that brought her feelings to the surface.

IT TAKES TIME

Getting over loss takes time; it is a gradual process. Feelings of sadness and emptiness do not suddenly disappear, never to return again. Rather, they diminish slowly, like wisps of fog burned off by the sun. Be gentle with yourself if it takes you longer to get over your loss than you think it should. Take whatever time you need. Give yourself permission to grieve; the loss of children *is* a profound loss.

Step 1 will be with you off and on for years, but as time passes, the intensity of the feelings will gradually diminish; the stimuli that evoke feelings of loss will decrease. Sorrow will change to sadness,

sadness to occasional wistfulness. What you are doing now—acknowledging that you will not have a child and letting yourself experience the loss—is the most painful part of resolution. It does get easier.

"Oh, the Loss, the Sorrow"

ANITA'S STORY

Anita's primary goal in life as a child and teenager was to be a wife and mother, like her own mother. One of three girls, Anita grew up in Seattle, where her father sold insurance. Not long after she married, at the age of nineteen, she learned that she was infertile. Anita is now fifty years old, and she readily admits the price she has paid for *not* acknowledging and experiencing her loss. Anita's defenses were so entrenched that she hardly dared discuss the issue: it took her five weeks of soul-searching before she decided to talk to me.

"It's been a silent nightmare for me. I was only twenty years old when the doctor first told me I would probably never get pregnant because of a congenital abnormality. I refused to believe it, and my husband couldn't deal with it either. We got a divorce a few years later, to the delight of my mother-in-law, who treated me like an outcast because I couldn't have children. I was so traumatized. I was ashamed that the marriage didn't work, ashamed that I didn't have children. I was a mistake as a person, useless as a person.

"I never said to anyone then, 'I'm never going to have any children.' I never said that out loud to anybody. I didn't say it to myself either. I couldn't. It just lay there. Years went by. I was so vastly alone with it. No one, not my mother, not my sisters, no one helped me. Why didn't someone say, 'Anita, you need to talk about this'? And it never dawned on me to get help.

"I didn't deal with anything. I hid because I was ashamed; I buried myself by going back to school and working nights. I backed away from my friends who were married and had children, because I couldn't bear their happiness. I've lost so much more than just my ability to have children. I've lost the growing-up years with those kids. They're all adults now.

"Every time somebody would have a baby I'd knit something. I had to do something with my hands. I can't explain what comfort there was in knitting, but I had to knit them all something. I must have knit country miles of baby clothes.

"I must have used a lot of energy in *not* dealing with it. Sometimes I can feel the pain well up from somewhere deep inside me, and I'll cry over the littlest things that don't mean anything. When I allow myself to talk about it, it gets to be so big, it's like some big mountain I can't get over. I'm afraid to let go, the floodgates will be so awful. I'm afraid I'll wear myself out with the tears. Oh, the loss, the sorrow!

"I just know there are whole parts of me not living because I've pulled away so badly. At least I know that now. Maybe that's the first step for doing something about it."

Anita and I met twice and talked for four hours. She cried most of the time. For the first time in thirty years she openly acknowledged her loss and allowed herself to experience it. After we talked, Anita decided to take a second step; she attended the wedding of a friend's daughter. Neither step was easy for her, but she has made a start.

"A Kiss on the Cheek"

CAROL'S STORY

Carol grew up in St. Louis. Her parents divorced when she was three, and she has never known her father. She has three sisters, two older, one younger. She dropped out of high school when she was sixteen. At nineteen she married a man ten years older than herself.

Carol has polycystic ovarian disease and has been told she cannot have children. Her husband already has children from a first marriage, and while he would like to have children with Carol, he refuses to consider adoption. Carol is twenty-two and drives a schoolbus in rural Missouri.

"I was always a dreamer, and I dreamed of marriage and children all the time. It meant the world to me to have a child to call my own. I always thought that having children was a big part of being a woman.

"It's been very hard for me to deal with. I cry a lot, feel sorry for myself. I feel like no one understands how I feel. It's like being in a room full of people and you're still alone. The pain for me is still real every time I see somebody with a baby. I cry for what will never be. They say time heals all wounds, but I think this is one wound that will never heal, no matter how much time passes.

"If you don't have children, people think you don't like kids or you're selfish and uncaring, that you don't want to tie yourself down. They don't ever think that maybe you just can't.

"I know I've missed a lot. I've missed the joy and happiness a child can bring to one's life. I'll never see my babies grow up. I'll never see them laugh or cry. I won't spend Christmas or vacation with them. I'll never have the pleasure of being called Mom. I won't have the closeness I wanted with my kids, like my mom had with me. Most of all, I realize I can never get or give such a simple thing as a kiss on the cheek from or to my children. I'm missing out on a very important part of my life. There will always be that empty space."

Carol *is* experiencing her loss fully. Difficult and painful as that is, it does mean that later, when the time is right for her, she will be able to take other steps toward resolution.

STEP TWO

Understanding the Loss

Rational, intellectual understanding helps an individual make sense of and communicate about her world. When experiences evoke painful, sometimes overwhelming emotions, as can happen with childlessness, a woman who can analyze a situation and identify its components has a decided advantage. Self-knowledge enables a woman to set her course through stormy seas when otherwise she might flounder.

If we feel intense emotions but do not know why, we experience a little epiphany, an "Oh, *that's* why I feel the way I do!" when we *do* figure out *why*. Understanding *why* brings relief and decreases our anxieties and frustrations by reassuring us that we are not going crazy or acting inappropriately.

Understanding in and of itself does not change behavior or feelings, however. You may know individuals, as I do, who have a thorough and correct understanding of why they have the problems they have. They can analyze the impact of early childhood experiences ad nauseam, or they can give a detailed, accurate assessment of their own personalities, yet they make no positive changes in their lives. But used correctly, as antecedents, not replacements for action, knowledge and understanding do aid resolution.

HIDDEN REASONS FOR WANTING CHILDREN

Gaining insight into the obvious, and the not so obvious, reasons why we wanted children helps us understand our loss. Often, though, we do not know why we wanted a child so intensely. Complex motivations influence much of human behavior, and the reasons we give ourselves for the ways we feel and act may not be the primary reasons at all. For example, a young woman who marries a man against her parents' wishes believes she does so *only* because she loves the man deeply. Many years later she may come to see just how much her choice of a mate was influenced by her need to assert her independence. Complex motivations also influence our longing for children. Sometimes we have hidden reasons, reasons that influence how we react to childlessness.

Many of us who feel traumatized when we do not have children are puzzled by the enormity of our reactions. We expect to feel some disappointment and sadness, but we are "blown away" by the intensity and force of our feelings. What we fail to understand is that childlessness triggers painful issues from other times or other areas of our lives. Thus we are dealing not only with the very real issue of wanting a child and not having one but also with other unresolved issues. I have seen individuals in therapy who come because they cannot get over the loss of a pet. "It's ridiculous," they might say. "I'm crying more now than I did when I lost my mother a year ago." The dynamic at work here is that one loss, the loss of a pet, reactivates previous losses that were never resolved. The grief in this instance is for *both* the pet and the mother, and possibly other unresolved losses as well. In the same way, the losses associated with childlessness can reactivate previous losses in a woman's life.

In the sections that follow, as you examine the less obvious reasons why women want children, you may worry that your reasons appear selfish, or you may feel guilty because you wanted children to meet your own needs. If so, do not judge yourself harshly. The *you* that you are today is the result of many influences in your life, sometimes powerful, negative influences you could not control or change as a child. Remember, the goal of this step is to increase your self-understanding, and you can do that best by accepting who you are instead of focusing on who you wish you were.

Psychological Reasons

To some extent, all parents experience their children as extensions of themselves. Given that children are flesh of our flesh, blood of our blood, that for nine months the developing fetus lies within the body of the mother, it is not surprising that women have a deeply embedded sense of the child as an extension of self. Identifying this dynamic helps us understand why a woman's unmet needs are often a powerful factor in her wish to have a child. Usually women are totally unaware that they hope to meet their needs vicariously through their children. This phenomenon does not occur only with women, of course; men too are often determined "to give the child every opportunity I didn't have." Since the child is seen as an extension of ourselves, it is as though whatever happens to our child happens to us too, to some degree.

Women who did not have loving, nurturing mothers when they were children dream of the day *they will be* loving, nurturing mothers to their own children. Always, they want to be better mothers than their own mothers were. It is as if they hope to reexperience the "good mother" by becoming the "good mother." As mothers, they would have control over the quality of the relationship in a way they did not have as a child. If a woman was never comforted and reassured when she was anxious and fearful as a child, she knows that it will be healing for her to comfort and reassure her own child.

When these women's longing for children goes unfulfilled, their inner child, still hungry for maternal love and nurturing, reexperiences loss all over again. This time it feels as though there is no hope to *ever* have the mothering they crave. A door has slammed in their faces; an opportunity for experiencing good mothering, albeit from the mothering end of the equation, is lost forever.

It may not be mothering that was lacking. The mother may have been perfectly adequate, but the father was cold and withdrawn or critical. Sometimes there was no father in the picture at all. Or both parents may have been loving toward the child, but their marital discord turned the home into a battleground. In these situations women want to recreate the family unit when they have children. They need to experience through families they create what they missed in their families of origin. If every holiday was ruined because the father drank and the parents fought when a woman was a child, then part of the reason she wants to make holidays warm and wonderful for her children is to heal her own wounds.

Few people have had perfect childhoods. Even given good-enough parents, life can be rough. Because we were not as smart or as cute or as talented or as rich or as popular as we wanted to be, a wounded inner child who still feels the hurts and humiliations of childhood and adolescence lies just beneath the surface for many of us. Parents, remembering their disappointments and embarrassments, hope to protect their children from similar hurts by providing the ballet lessons or the better clothes or the car or the college education or whatever it is they lacked as children. Of course, it does not work. Parents cannot shield children from the stings and heartaches of life. Parents cannot control the world and make everything right for their children. But children—including our own inner child—do not know that. When a woman hopes to exorcise some of her childhood pain through a better life for her children, her own inner child loses again when she remains childless. If her daughter is able to have a lovely new dress for her graduation dance, the woman no longer minds so much that she had to wear her sister's unfashionable hand-me-down dress to her own graduation dance.

SOCIAL REASONS

Sometimes our reasons for wanting a child have social origins. Like the woman who was told, "You won't be a woman until you have a child," many women see becoming a mother as a rite of passage. In our paternalistic society, mothers have been idealized and glorified—verbally, at least—and young women may feel that motherhood is the surest way to validate their worth and importance in others' eyes. In many families where sons are seen as being more important than daughters, where sons are seen as the ones who do exciting, interesting things in the world, a woman may want to have children because *she* holds center stage when she is expecting or has just given birth to a baby.

Any nonmother who has been present when mothers discuss their pregnancies, deliveries, and current experiences with children knows there is a special sisterhood that exists between women who have children. Motherhood confers the badge of membership, and childless women conspicuously lack the badge. Humans are social creatures; our well-being suffers when we feel excluded from the inner circle. Many childless women remark on the difficulty of establishing or maintaining friendships with women who have children, particularly when the children are young. The difficulty of holding a normal adult conversation, especially on the telephone, when children are present is one factor, as is finding common interests and conversational topics. As one woman jokingly said, "They don't want to hear about my cats; I don't want to hear about their children."

Children, especially babies, bring a lot of attention. People, even strangers, love to coo and cluck at babies. They love to smile and wave at toddlers. A mother with her baby or toddler holds center stage. Most humans like positive attention, so it is not surprising that mothers, especially women who receive little attention themselves, bask in the attention their children bring. Some shy women who are uncomfortable in social situations feel relief when attention shifts from them to the child. Childless women get neither the vicarious attention they desire nor, if they are shy, the welcome shift of attention away from themselves.

Women may also want children to save or cement relationships with men. Not that long ago, when men were pressured to marry a single woman whom they had impregnated, some women used pregnancy to hold onto the man they loved. Even today, without the social pressure, an unplanned pregnancy may propel a couple into marriage years before they would have married otherwise—if they would have married at all. More common, though, is the married woman who believes having a baby will save a shaky marriage. Children certainly provide a significant area of mutual interest in a marriage; unfortunately, that does not necessarily translate to a stronger marriage. If a couple fights about money and sex and friends, they will probably fight even more intensely about children.

Existential Reasons

Some women need children to give meaning and focus to their lives. These women find little genuine pleasure in their jobs, and their primary relationships, if any, are disappointing. Disillusioned with life itself, they just go through the motions. They may believe that their whole lives would turn around if only they had a child. Then they would have a noble reason for living. Their willing devotion to the child's well-being would provide meaning and purpose to life, a purpose beyond themselves. A child would fill the empty spots in their lives.

Loneliness is fertile ground for despair and desperation. Some women are lonely because they have no partners; others have partners who are not soul mates. Single women may have good friends who would be there for them immediately in a time of crisis, but they have no one to whom they are paramount on a day-to-day basis. These childless women often have the fantasy that they would not be lonely if they had children. Perhaps, in the early years of a child's life, before the child asserts independence, before the child develops friends and interests of her own, while the child still believes the sun rises and sets with Mommy, this fantasy may have some reality. Is there another human being who is loved and needed and desired as much as is a young child's mother? And so, some women long for children as an antidote for loneliness.

DIGGING DEEPER

Part I of this book identifies many losses childless women experience: loss of love, love that would have been given to a child, love that would have been received from a child; loss of friendship, especially with adult children; loss of support through an extended social network; loss of continuity of generations; loss of physical and developmental experiences.

You may already know what kind of loss you feel most deeply. If not, ask yourself the following questions. Why did I want children? What did I think children would add to my life? What is the hardest part for me about being childless? Be as specific as possible. Write down your responses and save what you have written.

Even if you think you have a good understanding of your obvious and/or hidden reasons for wanting children, you can learn more about yourself by answering the questionnaire you will find at the back of the book. These are the questions answered by women I interviewed or women who wrote to me. By looking at childlessness in the context of your total life, you will come to understand much more what having children means to you. Again, write down your responses and save them. When you work on Steps 7 through 10—rechanneling mothering energy, including children in your life, maximizing the advantages of childfree living, and embracing the quest for feminine wholeness, you will be ready to address your loss, ready to find new ways to meet your unmet needs. For now, identifying them is enough.

"Part of a Loving Family"

PAT'S STORY

Pat grew up in a university town in Montana. Both her parents, who are now dead, were alcoholics. She has one brother, but she and her brother are not close. Pat has been involved in numerous long-term relationships with men, none of which led to the marriage and family she desires. She is now thirty-five and works as an assistant manager at a bank.

"I always thought I would get married and have four children. I was going to have them one right after the other. And I had very clear ideas about how I would raise them. I would *not* bring them up with a negative focus like my parents brought me and my brother up with. My mother wasn't very happy being a mother, and it was clear to me that I didn't want to be like she was. She wasn't much fun to be around, and she constantly complained about her lot in life. We used to hear all year long about the money she spent on us at Christmas.

"I always wanted to experience that emotional bond of mothers with their children. I didn't have it with my mother, so it's hard for me to imagine what it's like. It must be a magnificent thing, powerful to feel so attached to someone. Not coming from a strong family, I thought I could experience that with my own family, with a generation I had created. I knew I could create a good family atmosphere if I had my own family.

"There was a time when I couldn't even watch 'The Waltons' on television because it used to make me cry. This was after I decided I couldn't hack it with my family, and I'd moved away. I'd see this warm, loving mother and father and all these children, and I realized there was never going to be a warm loving family for me—not when I was a child, not when I was an adult. That's what I've missed the most about being childless, the chance to be part of a loving family, my own loving family."

Women like Pat, who *never* have a chance to be part of a warm loving family, not when they are children, not when they are adults, help us understand why childlessness can be so devastating. It is sad enough to miss one of those experiences but heartbreaking to lose both.

"A Child in All of Us"

LAVERNE'S STORY

LaVerne was adopted as a baby and has always had a troubled relationship with her parents, especially her mother. She is divorced now but was married for twenty-three years to a man she describes as immature. She wanted children but felt she could not support her husband, financially and emotionally, *and* have a child. She is now fifty-three.

"I think a lot of healing happens in having children. There is a child in all of us, and to have a child is manifesting that on the outside. They *are* the inner child. They're the raw material. When we were children, we weren't really able to take care of ourselves, and now having a child enables us to take care of ourselves the way we wanted to be taken care of. We try to give our children what we didn't get.

"My mother bequeathed me a lot of her fears and shame and guilt about stuff that happened to her, things I didn't even know about until I was grown up. I think she got part of all that emotional garbage from her mother. What we don't work out, we pass down. But I think what hurt me the most was my parents' dishonesty. There was a lot going on between them, and I knew it because I was a sensitive person, but they would tell me it wasn't happening. They would be fighting, and I would say, 'Why are you mad at each other?' and they'd say, 'We're not mad. You must be imagining things.'

"It wasn't until late in life that I realized I wanted a child for all the wrong reasons: to replace the family I never had, to make me look good, to give me the sense of continuity I didn't have with my parents because I was adopted. Having a child meant becoming mature and being accepted by other women. I wanted my child to excel in one way or another, to be what I couldn't be. Being a mother was my one chance to do something worthwhile.

"Since I divorced my husband and moved away from my mother, life looks a lot better. I've worked hard to build a good life for myself. Even so, the feeling of not being vital to anyone is very big with me. Everything I have in my life, and really it's a lot, isn't enough. It's filler. It's too late now, but deep down I still feel that if I had had a child, my life would be complete."

LaVerne can clearly identify her complex reasons for wanting a child. She needed to heal her inner child; she wanted a child to make her look good and give her social standing when she felt she could not achieve that herself; having been adopted, she wanted to establish a family blood tie with her own children. Even though her life has improved over the last few years, she feels an emptiness in her life, an emptiness a child could fill.

STEP THREE

Surviving the Loss

Step 3 is critical because it is a step of hope. Now is the time, this is the place where you can change your basic mind-set about a life without children. Hopelessness can turn to hope, resignation to resolution. When we change our attitudes toward childlessness, we set the stage to change our feelings, change our lives.

If you are traumatized by your childlessness, you may have trouble believing that you can feel any differently than you do right now. At this moment, from the depths of your despair, you may be unable to envision a happy future for yourself. Such a restricted view is not surprising: at times of great sorrow and/or depression, people often cannot see beyond the feelings that threaten to engulf them. You may even identify with Rachel's cry, "Give me children, or else I die." But the reality is that no matter how bad you feel, you will *not* die. Depending on your age, you may well live another twenty, thirty, forty years without the child you desired. Fortunately, you do not have to feel this way for the rest of your life.

Perhaps you were never traumatized by childlessness. You may have resigned yourself to a life without children, but deep down you felt that your life would always be second rate. If so, this step brings hope for you too. You *can* create a rich, satisfying, challenging life, as many other childless women have done. You do not have to settle for second best.

CHOOSING ONE'S ATTITUDE

In his book *Man's Search for Meaning,* Viktor E. Frankl helps us see that we do have options, that we *can* choose how we respond to disappointments and tragedies. Frankl was imprisoned in a German concentration camp, and he observed how prisoners endured the unspeakable hardships. Some gave up; they could not face life as it was. Others withdrew into themselves. But there were those who walked through the camps comforting others, those who shared their last piece of bread. Frankl says, "They offer sufficient proof that everything can be taken from a man but one thing: the last of the human freedoms—to choose one's attitude in any given set of circumstances, to choose one's own way."

As a social worker, I have seen the many different ways individuals react to tragedies. Faced with blindness, confinement in a wheelchair, diagnosis of a terminal illness, some individuals react with dignity and a determination to make the most of their lives, whatever hardships confront them. Other individuals are unable to surmount their difficulties; preoccupied with the unfairness of life, they give up, thereby missing the richness life still offers.

Facing childlessness is no different. You have experienced a major disappointment, perhaps a trauma in your life. You did not have complete control over what happened to you, but you do have control over how you react. *You* will choose the attitude you carry with you for the rest of your life. *You* will choose the way you face it. You, I, each of us decides how we react to not having children. We are responsible, in the final analysis, for coming to terms with our disappointment, for resolving our loss. No one else can do it for us.

A WILLINGNESS TO MOVE ON

"But I don't know *how!*" you may protest. "Saying it won't make it so!" And you are absolutely right. Simply saying to yourself, "Okay, that's it, no more sadness, I'm going to get on with my life," will not make the bad feelings disappear. Life does not work that way.

Willing something to be so will not make it happen. But you must be willing for it to happen. I am reminded of something I once read about the pursuit of happiness: "You can't get there by trying, but you can't not try." Letting go of sadness and disappointment is like that. Just by *willing* it to be gone, you cannot make it so. But before it can happen, you must be open to the change; you must be willing to let go.

Although it sounds nonsensical, people sometimes cling to feelings of sadness and disappointment. There are various reasons why this is so. In the case of childlessness, you may feel that a willingness to move on implies that your wish for a child was trivial. After all, if you can get over it, how important could it have been? Or you may have grown so accustomed to feeling bad that it has become a part of you; you cannot even visualize yourself as a happy, satisfied person.

An element of self-love comes into play at this stage. Do you care enough about yourself that you are determined *not* to be unhappy for the rest of your life? Do you care enough about yourself that you are determined to create a rich, full, satisfying life for yourself, even though it will be a life without children? I am not suggesting that at this point in your resolution you know *how* to create that life. The how will come slowly, with time. But first must come the commitment to self. First must come the determination.

Some of you may have trouble making the commitment to a happier future. You find you have lost the habit of caring about yourself, or you feel you have no *right* to be happy. If so, you need to change the way you treat yourself, the way you view yourself. One helpful way to do this is to become your own best friend. One woman I know calls this her sitting-up-with-a-sick-friend routine. When she finds she is being hard on herself (for whatever reason), she pictures how she would treat a sick friend and tries to treat herself with the same kindness, gentleness, patience, and respect that she would extend to that friend. Tell yourself (even if you do not believe it at first), "I do deserve to be happy. I do deserve to have a good life. Others have gotten over this, and I can too."

If you find that negative feelings about yourself persist, I urge you to seek professional counseling. The losses of childlessness may be superimposed on and masking deep feelings of low self-esteem that have plagued you all your life. With professional help, you can change these negative feelings. You can find your way to a brighter future. With the right help, you will find that enormous changes are possible.

VICTIM OR SURVIVOR?

One woman I interviewed who had done rape counseling introduced me to the important concept of moving from a position of being a victim to that of being a survivor. When a woman has been raped, not surprisingly she feels like a victim. But victims are helpless and powerless; they cannot protect themselves or influence what happens to them. They are at the mercy of others. An important step in recovery takes place when a woman begins to see herself not as a victim but as a survivor, as someone who has faced adversity, survived it, and emerged stronger. Survivors are tenacious and resourceful people who rise above difficult circumstances.

So it is with childlessness. You may feel victimized because you were not able to have the child you wanted. Such feelings are real and valid, as all feelings are, but they are not helpful in resolving loss. Try reframing the way you see yourself. You faced a major disappointment in life, you survived it, and the future lies ahead, a future *you* can influence. If you start to think of yourself as a survivor, you will feel stronger, more in control, more able to face the future.

STRIVING FOR SERENITY

You may be familiar with the Serenity Prayer, which is an important part of the Alcoholics Anonymous Twelve-Step Program:

> God, grant me the serenity
> to accept the things I cannot change,
> the courage to change the things I can,
> and the wisdom to know the difference.

You cannot change the fact that you are childless. That is your reality; that is my reality. Whether we like it or not, we cannot change it. What we can change is how we perceive our childlessness and the effect it will have on the rest of our lives. If we have the courage and the will, we can reach for resolution. We *can* achieve serenity in our hearts and our lives.

"I Want to Be Happy"

JAMIE'S STORY

When she was nineteen, Jamie, who is now twenty-nine, fell in love with a man twenty-five years older than herself. She knew he did not want more children because his previous experience as a father had been a "nightmare," but she believed she could change his mind. She could not, and she was devastated when the man had a vasectomy shortly before they married. Although she loves her husband deeply and does not regret having married him, she longs to be a mother.

"When I married my husband, I truly believed that my maternal instinct would fade, but it didn't. It got stronger. For years, I felt so empty inside, so alone. I really felt like a mother with no baby. Every time I saw a pregnant woman, I wished it could be me. It was a pain that just wouldn't go away. I even thought of suicide.

"What changed everything for me was learning several months ago that I have malignant melanoma in my vaginal area. Somehow, being told I have cancer really helped me see the light. All those years I felt life wasn't worth living if I couldn't have a child, but now that I might die, I see how beautiful life is. I really feel that sadness and remorse can cause disease in our bodies. I just know that ten years of being depressed and wanting to die has helped to create cancer in my body.

"I used to blame myself and my husband, but now I see I can't undo the past. What's done is done. It won't be easy learning to accept being childless, but I'm trying to be positive about my life. I guess it's always easier to be unhappy. It takes a lot of work to be happy, and I see now that my happiness is up to me. I don't have a child, and it looks like I never will, but I want to be happy anyway. I want to be well."

When Jamie learned she had cancer, the diagnosis shocked her into a new perspective on her life. She had despaired about a future with no children, but now she realizes how much she wants a future. Changing our attitude helps us value our lives and frees us for new challenges.

"Do I Want to Accept It?"

MARJORIE'S STORY

Marjorie had parents who were loving to their four children but did not love each other. Marjorie's first marriage, which lasted twelve years, was tumultuous and consumed all her time and energy. She wanted children but did not want to bring them into an unhappy family. When she married her second husband—she was then forty—she tried to have a child. During the next four years Marjorie became pregnant twice, but she miscarried both times. She is now fifty.

"I went through the worst of my pain about being childless after the divorce. When I first confronted my childlessness, it was a horrible emotional experience. I'd say it is high on the list of the most painful things I've had to go through. But it was also a time of growth. I had been a real wimp during my marriage, and I learned to be an emotionally, mentally, and physically strong person.

"Then, in my second marriage, after the two pregnancies ended in miscarriages, I realized the deck was stacked against me, and I knew I had to make a decision. I asked myself, 'Do you want this to be the all-consuming, focal point of your life, or do you want to accept it?' I decided I had to learn to accept it. Acceptance doesn't mean the problem goes away. You have to continue to deal with whatever you're accepting. You don't resolve it once and it's forever, but it will come.

"I've had days when I feel depressed, defeated, and want to storm at the world, but that's very rare anymore. Sometimes I indulge in self-pity, but I think it's important not to make it a habit. I'm pretty good at taking something negative and using that energy for positive results. That's how I cope. I don't claim that my pain is gone, because I still have a feeling of wistfulness. But what is gone is the desire to have a child now.

"Another thing that helped me was that in other ways my life became very fulfilling. I've been busy working on myself, my life, my relationships. I've been actively creating my reality, pursuing my other dreams, and living where and how I want to live. I think it's important to take your energy and do something positive with it. Don't waste it. I'm now in an incredibly wonderful marriage, and I have stepchildren. My life now is very good, very fulfilled."

When Marjorie came face to face with the likelihood that she would never have children, she made a conscious decision to find some way to accept her childlessness. It was not easy, and it did not always work, but the alternative was a lifetime of disappointment and regret. Because Marjorie actively pursued other relationships and other interests, her life is now very satisfying.

STEP FOUR

Letting Go of Blame

Blaming seems to be an almost innate human quality. Young children learn to blame at an early age, soon after speech develops. They blame their siblings, their friends, the dog, the cat—whoever is handy. As they get older they also learn—some too well—to blame themselves.

None of us is perfect; we do make mistakes. If we are to learn from our mistakes, we must identify which of our attitudes and behaviors brought about the problem. *This* part of blame, identifying and assuming responsibility, can be a positive growth experience. It is the other part of blame, the expression of disapproval or reproach, the censure, that so often acts as a negative force in our lives.

Preoccupation with any negative emotion—jealousy, hatred, blame—poisons our lives. Inevitably, negative feelings harm the individual who feels them far more than they harm the individual to whom they are directed. When the two, subject and object, are one and the same, namely, ourselves, the damage is compounded. When we hold onto blame, we anchor ourselves firmly in the past. It is only when we let go of blame that we free ourselves to move forward.

Blame can be rational or irrational and often has elements of both. The intensity of blame has little to do with the existence or lack of rational reasons. Irrational blame can be just as intense as rational blame, and it is often more difficult to deal with, because it springs not from exterior causes but from unfathomable sources deep within ourselves.

WHOM WE BLAME

Ourselves tops the list of those we blame the most. We blame ourselves for

- being unable to conceive
- having miscarriages
- having imperfect bodies
- having abortions
- postponing a decision about having children
- falling in love with and marrying partners who do not want children
- agreeing to childlessness without really thinking through what that means
- connecting with the wrong men
- putting men's needs ahead of our own
- not being "together enough" or not getting our lives "together enough" to marry and have children

Husbands and partners take second place as the people most often blamed. We blame them for

- having fertility problems
- not wanting children
- not wanting more children
- not being willing to adopt
- not being willing to try donor insemination
- insisting on abortions
- postponing a decision about having children
- being poor father material because they are immature, are on drugs, drink excessively, gamble, etc.
- not understanding how much a child means to us

Parents occasionally get blamed as well. We blame parents for

- raising us in dysfunctional families, thereby depriving us of the mental health and maturity we needed to marry and have children of our own
- passing their pathology on to us
- pressuring us to have abortions
- programming us to be career women (so we would never be trapped as our mothers had been)

Mothers-in-law may not be responsible for our childlessness, but we blame them for

- rejecting us when we could not have children

Our stepchildren's biological mothers get blamed for

- raising their children in a way we do not like

- upsetting our husbands and interfering in our lives
- setting our stepchildren against us

Doctors and medical staff are blamed for

- treating us in a cavalier manner
- being insensitive to our needs, both physically and emotionally
- putting us through painful procedures and tests and acting as though we should not mind the pain

God or fate is blamed because

- God can do anything; God could have given us a child
- we have no one else to blame

Adoption agencies are blamed for

- having ridiculous criteria for suitable adoptive parents, criteria that exclude us because we are not married or we are too poor or our bathrooms are too small

WHY WE BLAME

We blame because we are angry that we do not have children. Anger needs, it seeks, a target. Unfocused, free-floating anger frustrates us more than does focused anger. Having a target for our anger makes an undesirable situation more tolerable. When we think we know who is to blame, we feel justifiable outrage and moral indignation. When we focus on the target of our blame, we forget, at least momentarily, our loss and our sadness.

A second reason why we blame, a deeper and more intriguing reason, is based on the common belief that a problem is easier to solve if we know what caused it. If we can find a concrete, readily identifiable reason why we do not have children, then there is the very real possibility of finding a remedy and reversing the situation—at least that is what our illogical hearts want to believe.

One woman we have already met, Jeanne, who had had multiple miscarriages, continues to blame herself for doing something wrong. (You will remember that she did not know what she had done wrong, but she thought perhaps she was not relaxed enough or had walked too fast or should not have had sex.) During our talks together, we explored her tenacious, intractable self-blame—which she knows is irrational—and tried to make sense of it. "I know what it is," she finally whispered. "You see, if I did something wrong, maybe I can figure out what it was, and *then* I can do it right and I'll have a baby. Otherwise, if I'm *not* to blame, if I'm not responsible, there's no hope. Then I have to accept that I'll never have a child." No wonder she clings to self-blame; it is her lifeline to hope, an irrational lifeline, but a lifeline nonetheless.

If you use blame like Jeanne does, you may have to deliberately extinguish all hope of ever having a child—painful as that will be—in order to free yourself of blame. Neither blame nor hope can undo the past, and clinging to false hope will not enrich the present or the future.

ACCEPTING RESPONSIBILITY FOR THE PART WE PLAYED

Most of us have played some part in our childlessness. I know I certainly did. If you search your heart and examine your life, you will probably find that you, too, perhaps unintentionally, made decisions that contributed to your being childless. You may have had an abortion. You may have chosen and stayed with a partner who did not want children. You may have decided not to be a single mother. You may have decided not to adopt. Identifying the part we played helps us relinquish the blame we direct at others. If you have not previously considered the role you played, now is the time to do so.

Identifying and accepting my own responsibility (with the help of a supportive, competent therapist) was an important step for me. I saw that I had contributed to my childlessness because I acquiesced to my ex-husband's ambivalence. I could have insisted we have a child; I could have stopped using birth control and not told him (as many women do when their partners do not want children); I could have left him. I did none of those things, and so I too played a role, albeit unwittingly, in causing my childlessness. Later, when my present husband and I could not have children because of infertility problems, I chose not to adopt because I had neither the energy nor the will for more uncertainty and dashed hopes.

When you first see that you did play a part, you may turn on yourself the anger and blame that you used to direct at others. I suppose it is natural to do so. I certainly went through a period during which I blamed myself. Fortunately, my self-blame was short lived, perhaps because my background as a social worker has shown me that there are legitimate reasons why people act the way they do, why they make the decisions they make, though the reasons may not be known or understood by the people themselves. Seemingly illogical behavior makes sense only when viewed in the total context of an individual's life.

For example, many women's need for psychological security is so tied in to parents (when we are younger) and to partners (when we are older) that we cannot risk asserting ourselves and our own needs. It can feel as though our very survival depends on the relationship, and the relationship in turn may seem to depend on our meeting others' needs or gaining their approval. Given the high stakes, our course of action (or inaction) makes sense.

If you want to ferret out your deeper reasons for certain behaviors or decisions, try the following: take a respectful attitude toward yourself; assume there *are* legitimate reasons why you did what you did, reasons that make sense, given your life experiences; suspend judgment; do not censure your responses; and then say to yourself, "I did ——— because ———." Often a deeper psychological reason will emerge. I know that gaining a better understanding of myself helped me accept responsibility without blame.

Abortions

Of all the many actions women take and the decisions they make as they travel the varied paths that lead to childlessness, having chosen to have an abortion is the one that can most readily lead to self-blame. The woman has conceived; she is pregnant. The odds are that if she does nothing she will have a child. Usually a woman assumes, reasonably enough, that she will have other pregnancies, that she will have children later. After all, many women who had abortions do have children. When this does not happen, a woman may blame herself for having deliberately ended a pregnancy. And then again she may not.

Many women I interviewed had had abortions, and their reactions to those abortions fit into three main categories:

1. *Women who are at peace with the decision they made and would make the same decision again.* A number of women did not blame themselves. They understood that, given the circumstances of their lives at the time of the abortion, they did what they had to do. They may regret those circumstances, and they certainly regret not having children, but they do not blame themselves for having had an abortion. One woman said, "My husband was very young, and he couldn't have handled a baby then. I loved him very much, and I'm sure I'd do the same thing again if I were in the same situation. I don't blame myself for the abortion. I'm just sorry I wasn't able to

have children later." Another woman said, "I wanted a baby very much, but not as a single mother. I still don't want that, so it was the right decision. I did what I had to do."

2. *Women who regret that they had abortions but do not blame themselves.* These women say that if they had been able to see into the future (their childless future), they would *not* have had an abortion. Even so, even though they regret what they did, they do not blame themselves. "I did what I thought was the best thing at the time. You can't do more than that," one woman said. Another told me, "You can go crazy if you start examining your life in terms of 'What if I'd done this instead of that?' You can really drive yourself crazy. Who needs it?"

3. *Women who do blame themselves because they had abortions.* These women are consumed with regret; they torment themselves with self-blame. They cannot find in their hearts, nor can they extend to themselves, even an ounce of mercy. "I'll never forgive myself for having had an abortion," one woman wrote. "I threw away my one chance to have a baby." "God is punishing me because I killed my baby," another woman said. While the remorse these women feel is understandable, it will not change the past, only rob them of the energy and the perspective needed to move on and build a worthwhile life. Fortunately, these intense feelings of blame *can* change. Women do learn to forgive themselves with the help of therapy, spiritual pursuits, and self-help groups.

DYSFUNCTIONAL FAMILIES

One other category of women who tend to be very hard on themselves is women who grew up in severely dysfunctional families. Their self-blame now echoes the negative messages they received all their lives. While some of these women wanted children and decided not to have them because they were determined *not* to pass along the pathology, most had longed to experience in families they formed what they had not experienced in their families of origin. "I feel like I'm a failure because I could never get my act together enough to do the usual bit of marriage and children," one woman said. "I wanted it, but it was always out of reach." Hearing their life stories, I was astonished at what they *had* achieved, against all psychological odds. They had careers that satisfied them immensely, and some had happy marriages.

If you grew up in a dysfunctional family and blame yourself for being childless, maybe you need to step back and take a fresh look at what you *have* done with your life. Given that you are an ordinary mortal, not a mythic heroine who can surmount any obstacle and slay any dragon in her path, if you are not addicted to drugs or alcohol, if you are not suicidal, to name extreme examples, you should congratulate yourself. Yes, if things had been different you would have liked to have children, but things were not different. Give yourself credit for what you have done.

It also helps to try to understand what made your parents who they are. Often they too grew up in dysfunctional families, but with the added misfortune of doing so at a time when there was less help available and people had less understanding of psychological needs. Usually parents do the best they can for their children, though their vision of what is best may have evolved by their looking through woefully distorted lenses. Understanding your parents will not change the wounding that has taken place, but knowing that they too had their problems to contend with, that they did not begin parenthood with a blank slate, will help.

HOW TO STOP BLAMING

The following exercises, adapted here for our purposes, are frequently used in therapeutic growth-oriented sessions. When you use them, you need to adopt the same supportive, gentle attitude we talked about in Step 3 when I described the advantages of adopting a helping-a-sick-friend approach toward yourself. The more understanding and comfort you can offer to yourself, the better.

Writing Forgivenesses

A powerful written exercise that I have found to be very helpful, not only in regard to childlessness, is the exercise of writing forgivenesses. In one sentence summarize who and what it is that needs forgiving and write that sentence twenty times. (The "who" may be yourself or someone else; see below for examples.) The next day construct another sentence that expresses how you feel then, and write it twenty times. Do not worry if what you are writing is not a true reflection of how you feel. The statement is one of intention, and repetition helps to make the intention reality. If you do the exercise consistently, you will find that anger and blaming diminish. The exercise helps to clean old angers and resentments out of the system. Here is an example:

> Day 1: I, Marie, forgive my mother for being insensitive and selfish and forcing me to have an abortion. (Repeat twenty times.)
>
> Day 5: I, Marie, forgive my mother for not understanding how much I wanted a baby and for pressuring me to get an abortion. (Repeat twenty times.)
>
> Day 10: I, Marie, forgive my mother for doing what she thought was best. (Repeat twenty times.)

If you are working on forgiving yourself, the sentences might be

Day 1: I, Marie, forgive myself for waiting too long to marry and have children.

Day 5: I, Marie, forgive myself for not following through on adopting a child.

Day 10: I, Marie, forgive myself for being afraid to be a single mother.

HAVING A DIALOGUE WITH THE PERSON YOU BLAME

This exercise will be helpful whether you blame yourself or others. You do it by yourself, taking both parts of the dialogue. You may do it either in writing or by talking to yourself aloud. (Dialogues in your head do not have the same effect.) Some people who dialogue out loud find it helpful to use two chairs and change seats, depending on which part of themselves or which person in a relationship is talking. Two condensed examples of how such a dialogue might go follow.

CRITICAL SELF: I'm such an idiot. I should never have agreed to Tom's vasectomy. Now I've cheated myself out of ever having a child. I'll never forgive myself. Or him.

FORGIVING SELF: You did have a reason.

CRITICAL SELF: Tom was so adamant about not wanting more children. If I hadn't agreed, I would have lost him, and I love him.

FORGIVING SELF: What a difficult choice! It makes me sad to see you faced with a choice like that.

CRITICAL SELF: It makes me sad, too.

FORGIVING SELF: I forgive you for what you did. It sounds like you couldn't have won whichever way you went. I wish you weren't so hard on yourself. You're not a bad person. You did what you thought was right.

CRITICAL SELF: No, I'm not a bad person. And neither is Tom. I understand his point of view, too. Life is just so damn difficult sometimes.

YOU: You know, Tom, sometimes I almost hate you for insisting on the vasectomy. You cheated me out of having a child. Sometimes I wonder if you really love me.

TOM: I *do* love you. I didn't know it would be this difficult for you. Why didn't you tell me?

YOU: Because I didn't know either! You just kept insisting and insisting. I was afraid I'd lose you.

TOM: And I was afraid of what having children would do to us.

YOU: To us? Or to you?

TOM: Okay, if I'm honest, what it would do to me. I raised one family, and it wasn't much fun. I could hardly wait until the time when *I* could have a life. And then I met you and knew I wanted you in that life. We can have a wonderful life. I know we can. You used to want that too.

YOU: I *do* want it too. But I have a lot of sadness about not having children. I need you to understand that and comfort me.

TOM: I do understand your sadness. I love you so much, and I want you to be happy. I really am sorry this has brought you so much unhappiness.

I REFUSE

Another written exercise that may help if you find your blaming is completely intransigent and refuses to budge is the "I refuse" exercise. When I get stuck, I often use this exercise to get a deeper understanding of the personal dynamics that are keeping me stuck. Do not be surprised if this exercise ties into something you learned about yourself in Step 2.

Without stopping to decide whether or not what you write makes sense, use the following sentence and write down the first ten things that come to mind: I refuse to stop blaming because ———.

SYMBOLIC CREMATION

My husband and I have a friend who belongs to a men's club that holds an annual two-week encampment in a lovely grove of redwood trees in northern California. Each year, at the beginning of the encampment, each member makes a list of all his cares, all the worries and sorrows that burden his life and his heart. For example, I am worried that business has dropped off; I am concerned about my son, who dropped out of college; I worry about the chest pains I am having. When the list is complete, a "Cremation of Care" ceremony is held, and the lists are burned, the cares symbolically cremated, the men symbolically set free.

Try this exercise on blame. Make a list of all the wrongdoings you can think of, either your own or those of others, everything that kept you from having a child. For example, I blame my parents for talking me into having an abortion when I was in high school; I blame myself for going along with them when I did not really want to; I blame myself for not being able to get pregnant now; I blame my husband for not wanting to adopt. Study your list and make sure it is complete. Keep it for a few days, if that feels right, and then burn it.

When we blame, we assume that the other path, the path not taken, would have been better. Perhaps it would have been, but no one can predict what your life would have been like if you, or someone else, had made different decisions. In all likelihood your life would not have been as rosy as you picture it in your fantasies: it would have had its own set of problems.

Be willing to let go of blame. It will pollute your life if you let it. Remember the oft-quoted (and here adapted) adage: to blame is human, to forgive divine.

"I Didn't Have It Within Me"

GAYLE'S STORY

Gayle, whose mother was repeatedly hospitalized for depression, grew up in a dysfunctional family and has also struggled with depression all her life. She married at twenty-three, and she and her husband now own and run a thriving travel agency. Both of them wanted a family, but Gayle kept postponing pregnancy because it was never the right time. In her early forties she realized she was running out of time, and she stopped using birth control. She soon became pregnant.

"I was always being teased as a child and didn't know how to handle it. I was self-conscious and awkward, very unhappy and very stubborn. The family was not poor, nor were we rich. I remember my mother telling me once that we were from the wrong side of the tracks. She never encouraged me in anything and constantly criticized me. My father was very remote. You could say I grew up with an inferiority complex.

"Not long after my husband and I married, he wanted to start a family, but I wasn't ready then. I was bored with being a housewife, and I didn't want to be stuck at home all my life like my mother had been. So we waited. After we started our business, it seemed like the time was never right. When I reached forty, I realized it was now or never.

"My husband was out of the country for a month when I got the news I was pregnant. Even though it was something I wanted, I was terrified. It's difficult for me to explain my fear; it was so irrational. I was afraid the child would be abnormal. I was terrified that I would die in childbirth. I was certain that I couldn't cope if I did survive. Later I found out that hormonal changes take place in pregnancy. Maybe that's why I panicked; I don't know. All I could think of was an abortion.

"I felt I couldn't talk on the telephone to my husband about the pregnancy or my reaction to it. The psychiatrist I was seeing was no help at all; he more or less told me it was my decision. I did have an abortion and regretted it from the time I dragged myself home from the clinic. I went into a very deep depression. I was incapacitated. I've blamed myself ever since. I feel so guilty. It was years before I could tell my husband about it. He forgave me, but he was disappointed. That's the hardest part for me; I blame myself because my husband doesn't have the children he always wanted."

When I talked to Gayle, four years after she had the abortion, I explained that sometimes people do have sound reasons why they do the things they do, survival reasons they are not aware of, and I asked what her reason might be. This was her answer. "I think I would have been overwhelmed. Maybe I didn't have it within me to care for someone else when it was all I could do to care for myself." Given Gayle's history, I think she was right. None of her siblings have managed to establish happy marriages or careers, and none of them have children. Gayle *does have* a good marriage, and she *does have* a rewarding career, both major achievements. Perhaps intuitively she knew what was right and appropriate for her.

"This Is Who I Am"

DOROTHY'S STORY

Although Dorothy always had female friends, her extreme shyness around boys and men meant she had few dates as an adolescent and young adult. In fact, she never had a significant emotional relationship with a male. A crippling car accident when she was forty-two brought an abrupt end to her career as a pediatric nurse. She now lives with her parents in her small hometown in Oklahoma.

"I've always wanted to marry and have children. When I worked as a nurse, it would break my heart when I cared for children who had been abused or emotionally damaged by their parents. I would grieve that I didn't have children or that I couldn't take those children and raise them the way they should be raised. I'd think, 'Oh, I would be such a good mother.' And then, when I was injured, the focus changed. My goal was to walk, to get better.

"It bothered me more when I was younger. I didn't ever cry about it. I didn't discuss it with people. It was a silent mourning. Once in a while I'll still have a pang about being childless. It's not depression, just a passing sadness. There's a time in your life when you could raise children, and then when you pass that time you realize it.

"Sometimes I've thought that if I could live my life over, I'd make more of an effort to meet guys in my early life. But if I'm really honest, I probably would have made the same choices again. I wouldn't have done anything differently. This is who I am. I've learned to accept that I played a part in how my life turned out. And I don't blame myself for being who I am.

"My cousin once said to me, 'Why don't you just get serious about this; I'm sure you'd get married, if you did.' I was serious, but you can't let that dominate you. I see myself as normal, but when I meet new people and they find out I'm not married and that I live with my parents, I can tell they think, 'Oh, strange lady.' I even get comments from people in my church that indicate they don't see me as normal. But it doesn't bother me. I may be different, but different isn't bad.

"My sister has a three-year-old, and we really love each other. She's at that stage where she classifies people. The other day she said, 'Mommy's a mother, grandmother's a mother, and you're a mother.' I said, 'I'm not a mother; I'm your aunt.' She looked really hurt, so I explained that I didn't have any children. 'Well, me,' she said. It really touched me. I thought, 'Well, I do have meaning in my life when I can relate to other children and they love me this much.'"

Dorothy deserves credit for understanding and accepting who she is. She knows that if, as a younger woman, she had been able to meet a man and marry, her life would have more closely approximated the life she wanted. But as she says, candidly, "I am who I am." All of us can say the same; we are who we are. If we were to relive our earlier lives, we would find ourselves doing the very same things once again, because we would have the same needs, the same inhibitions, the same situations we had then.

STEP FIVE

Talking to Significant Others

"No man is an island, entire of itself," John Donne wrote in 1624, and what he says of men is also true for women. One of our great strengths as women is our need for other people. Throughout our lives we turn to others for understanding, support, wisdom, and perspective. We use our relationships with significant other people to help us deal with the everyday challenges of our lives and with the crises that occasionally threaten to overwhelm us. Our wish to have children, to be mothers, lies so near the core of our being that, whether resolution is an everyday challenge or a crisis for us, it is a time when we need other people. Any sorrow, any disappointment can be borne more easily when we know others understand our feelings, when we know others care.

In addition to support and understanding, we also need the perspective other people can give. When all our thoughts and feelings are indwelling, we lose perspective. We go round and round in circles, seeing no solutions, thinking no new thoughts. Exposing our feelings and thoughts to the fresh air opens up our horizons and ends our circular absorptions. The feedback, advice, encouragement, and wisdom of others shed new light, bring new perspective to our situation.

Many times we benefit most not from what others say but from what we hear ourselves say. Talking to others is a powerful way to clarify our own thoughts and feelings. On a number of occasions I did not realize that I knew what to do about a certain situation until I heard what I said to someone else, things I knew but did not know I knew.

Some individuals respond to personal pain and pressure by withdrawing into themselves. They hope to protect themselves from further hurt by locking the doors and pulling up the drawbridge. Women who respond to childlessness in this way often find they have isolated themselves from many of the good things in life. Like Anita, whom we read about in Step 1, they avoid holiday gatherings, parties, office functions—any event where children may be discussed or will be present. By doing so, these women cut themselves off from the very interactions that would eventually ease their loss. It is difficult after any significant loss to embrace the fullness of life, to maintain contact with other people, to participate in social gatherings, but doing so is a potent antidote to loss.

THE DIFFICULTIES OF TALKING TO OTHERS

While there are exceptions, most childless women do not share their feelings of sadness, disappointment, and loss with other people. Throughout my research for this book, I was struck time and again by how few women had ever opened their hearts to anyone on this subject. Over and over again women told me, "I've never talked to anyone but you about how I feel." Women who talk to sisters, friends, and mothers about problems in marriages, traumatic experiences in childhood, or disappointments in their careers say, with few exceptions, that they *do not* talk about being childless. I interviewed two women who are best friends, both of whom had wanted to have children, both of whom talked to me frankly about their experiences and feelings, yet neither one had ever "really" talked to the other about being childless.

When women have discussed the subject with others, they have usually communicated on a superficial level, indicating they would have liked to have a child but in no way giving a true indication of the depth and complexity of their feelings. This is one reason why most people do not appreciate the numbers of women who longed to have children, why few people know how lingering and pervasive their disappointment is. *Women, by and large, have not talked about the experience of permanent childlessness.*

WHY WOMEN DO NOT SHARE

The primary reason we childless women do not share our feelings on this subject is, I believe, because we feel so terribly vulnerable. The vulnerability comes from two main sources. As we saw in Step 2, the child we wanted is often symbolic of our own inner child. When we talk about being childless, we are also talking about (and thus exposing) our own inner child, the most tender part of ourselves. The more vulnerable the inner child, the more a woman has been hurt by experience, the stronger is her need for safety. If she does not talk, if she remains silent, she guards the inner child. She remains safe.

The other main source of vulnerability is the inextricable link between mothering and our feminine identity. If we feel that we are not "real" women, or that we are "less than" other women, because we do not have children, we will go to great lengths *not* to publicly expose our inadequacy and inferiority. If we were to *really* discuss what mothering means to us, it would feel as though we had offered up our vital organs for examination and dissection. The subject is so sensitive that we may fear we will be unable to control our emotions and burst into tears. No one likes to appear foolish.

Social considerations are also a factor. Women do not talk because they fear social censure. Because the dominant cultural expectation is that women *will* marry and have children, some people value a woman more highly if she has children, just as they accord a woman higher status if she is married. For other women it is a matter of pride; they do not want to be objects of pity. Better to put on a brave front and keep one's feelings to oneself than risk the overheard whisper, "Poor Mary. She wasn't able to have children."

Sometimes women do not speak freely because they do not want to rain on someone else's parade. If you have a friend or sister or neighbor who is happily engaged in mothering, you may be reluctant to share your sadness because you do not want to inhibit her spontaneous sharing. You do not want to make her self-conscious when she talks about her children and the satisfaction she gains from mothering. If she monitors everything she says because she knows the subject is a tender, hurtful one for you, the relationship will suffer.

OTHERS WILL NOT UNDERSTAND

Women may choose not to confide in others because they fear others will not understand how they feel. Often they are right. Many women told me of insensitive remarks made by otherwise sensitive people. Sometimes the offenders are other childless women. One woman tried to talk about her sadness to her best friend, a single, childless woman. The friend's response, "But not everyone gets to be a mother," stated the obvious but was not a compassionate response to the woman's feelings at the moment. Women who are mothers, including childless women's own mothers, may respond by saying, "Be glad you don't have children; you don't know how lucky you are." Perhaps they hope to give comfort by focusing on the difficulties of being a mother, but childless women feel patronized by the casual dismissal of the subject. They know these women treasure their children, even though the children drive them crazy at times.

What childless women need when they share their feelings is to have those feelings validated. The following responses—"That must be difficult," "I feel for you," "I'm sorry you're so sad," "I'm glad you told me how you feel"—all communicate that the listener heard what the woman said and cares about her feelings. Women who share their troubles or heartaches with others do not expect their problems to be solved, nor do they want a pep talk. What they want and need is for their confidante to listen to and empathize with the feelings they express.

OTHER PEOPLE'S REACTIONS

Two factors influence how objectively, or emotionally, people react to a situation. One factor is the sensitivity of the subject. Most people can objectively discuss a remote issue, such as national legislation that proposes to change the amount of funding states receive for new highways. They find it more difficult to objectively discuss an issue that affects them directly, such as the installation of parking meters in a small town. The second factor that influences how people react is whether or not the subject is relevant to someone they care about. If we do not personally know anyone who is developmentally disabled, we will tend to talk objectively about a cut in funding for services to such people; if we have a sister who will no longer be able to attend the sheltered workshop that is the center of her universe, we tend to talk more emotionally. Your childlessness is a sensitive issue for those who care about you; do not be surprised if their reactions sometimes miss the mark.

When talking to close family members—husbands, parents, brothers, sisters—remember that they have their own feelings of sadness, disappointment, anxiety, and guilt about your childlessness. They may be preoccupied with their own concerns. A partner who wanted a baby may be struggling with feelings of loss because there will be no child. A partner who feels responsible for your happiness may be overwhelmed by your sorrow. Parents often feel tremendous sadness for their daughters. Because you are special to them, they may have longed to have a grandchild (your child), even though they have other grandchildren.

The more intense the feelings and reactions of others, the more difficult it is for them to respond to *your* needs. Partners, parents, and significant others in our lives may feel deeply for us but say nothing or say the wrong thing, either because they are trying to deal with their own feelings or because they do not know what to say.

If you confided your deep longing for a child to others, and over many years they shared your ups and downs from infertility studies or multiple miscarriages or attempts to adopt a child, they may have an emotional investment in your getting the child you want. When you do decide you have had enough, they may have trouble letting go. Several women mentioned this problem. One woman had talked to two close women friends about her husband's reluctance to try donor insemination when that was the last thing left to try. She finally decided she would not endanger the marriage over this issue, but her friends pressured her not to "give in" to her husband; they felt she deserved a baby. Another woman who married a man with teenage children found that he had invested so strongly in her dream to have a child that he could not let go when she was ready to end the years of infertility treatments. He kept urging her to try more and more procedures at a time when she wanted to make her peace with childlessness and move on.

Sometimes other people who have no idea why a woman is childless will pressure her to have children. Older brothers, well-meaning aunts and uncles, or parents take it on themselves to dispense pep talks about the joys of mothering. "You should start a family right away," they urge, oblivious to the sensitive feelings on which they tread. They want to help, they try to help, by sharing their perspective on the value of having children. What they fail to see is that they are preaching to the converted.

GUIDELINES FOR TALKING TO SIGNIFICANT OTHERS

Because childlessness is such a vulnerable subject and because there are dangers inherent in opening your heart to others, the choice of confidante(s) is extremely important. *Choose carefully the people with whom you share.* You do not need more heartache in your life; you do not need your tender feelings stomped on. *Test the waters first: start with a neutral, leading remark or question instead of jumping in with your heart exposed.* It is safer to say, "A neighbor of mine told me she's just found out she can't have children," than it is to say, "I'm really sad and depressed because I don't have children." See what kind of response the other person gives before you make yourself vulnerable.

Another helpful technique is to tell people what you need from them. Dialogue always has a greater chance of succeeding if the people involved each know what the other needs, wants, and expects from the conversation. If you know—and you may not—what it is you need, tell the other person. Is it understanding, advice, problem-solving techniques, a new perspective? It is helpful to say things like,

"I need a shoulder to cry on," "I need to share my sadness with you and know you understand," "I'm trying to come to terms with not having children, and I'm wondering if you'd share how you dealt with that issue."

I often recommend this technique when I do marriage counseling, and it is not unusual for one partner (often the woman) to discount this approach. "It doesn't mean anything if I have to ask for it," they will say. They mistakenly think that the compliment "you look nice" or the declaration "I love you" or whatever it is they need to hear is not sincere if it is given after being requested. We would all love for special people in our lives to say all the right things at all the right times, but that does not happen. Well-meaning, loving, sincere people often *do not know* what to do or say. Remember, the person you are talking to is not a mind reader. He or she does not automatically know what you need. The more guidance you can give, the more likely you are to receive what you need.

If you have people in your life who continue to pressure you or people who are nosy, a predetermined strategy may help. If you are willing to share your feelings or provide information about your situation, honesty can be highly disarming: "I feel bad that I don't have children, and I get sad every time the subject is brought up" should silence almost anyone. If people press for details, tell them, "You know, I really don't wish to discuss it."

If you do not want to tell people anything about your situation, you will need to be even more assertive: "Why do you ask?" is always an effective rejoinder. As an alternative, "I've always thought the subject of having children is a very personal one, don't you?" should work, followed by "I really don't wish to discuss it," if necessary. One woman got so fed up with her older brother's exhortations on the subject that she finally confided in a whisper, "I wanted to have children, but I have female problems that prevent it." He never brought the subject up again. Another woman noticed that whenever she and her mother were alone, her mother gently nudged the conversation toward the topic of having children. The woman decided to share the news that she had seen an infertility specialist. The mother then confided that she had had similar problems when she was young, and she provided enormous support to her daughter from then on.

Many childless women dread being asked, "Do you have children?" Remember that people who innocently ask this question have no way of knowing that the subject may be sensitive for you. The question *is* accepted in our culture as a legitimate way to learn more about people we meet, and it will come up over and over again. Try to prepare a response that defuses the question for you and for the person asking it. One woman I interviewed had found the perfect rejoinder. When asked if she had children, she replied, "No, but I have a demanding cat."

We women who wanted children live in the real world, not in a vacuum. Those people nearest and dearest to us will be touched by our childlessness in one way or another. If we find safe ways to share our feelings and experiences, if we reach out to others, if we tell them what we need, we benefit from their love, their concern, their wisdom. It is worth the risk.

"They Mean Well"

CHRISTIANA'S STORY

We heard from Christiana in Part II when relationship issues were explored as a reason for childlessness. Christiana is the woman who felt she had made "absurd choices."

"I have a sister who is ten years older than I am and a brother thirteen years older, and they've always thought they knew what was best for me. Usually it's amusing, but all of a sudden they both started pressuring me about having a baby.

"My sister would actually send children's books and clothes. 'For when you have your baby,' she'd write. My brother's a psychiatrist, so he should know better, but one day he telephoned and out of the blue started in on me. 'You've got to get serious about getting married and starting a family,' he said. 'You're thirty-four years old, and if you don't do something soon, it'll be too late.' He kept going on and on. Here he was, totally oblivious to the fact that he was stomping around on my most sensitive feelings. I mumbled something and hung up. I was totally stunned.

"But I was also furious. I thought of writing a scathing letter, but then I decided against it. I know they mean well. They really care about me. So I wrote them each a really frank letter and said, 'Look, can't you see there's nothing I want more than to marry and have children, but it hasn't happened for me? I appreciate your concern, but what I need is your understanding, not pressure. This is a very sensitive subject for me.'

"My sister called right away and apologized for pressuring me. She was very empathetic, and we had a heart-to-heart talk. Since then my brother has stopped the pressure too. Somehow he seems more tender toward me now. They still introduce me to available men when I visit, but I can put up with that. They mean well."

Christiana's gamble in openness paid off. By sharing her wish for a child and her sadness because she does not have one, she gained the understanding and concern of both her brother and sister. They no longer see her as a career woman who simply does not care about a husband and family, and she no longer sees them as insensitive and interfering.

"He Looked So Sad"

ISABEL'S STORY

We also heard from Isabel in Part II in the section on problem pregnancies. She is the woman who described herself as having "so many missing parts" after her two ectopic pregnancies.

"Interestingly enough, my father is the one person who seems to understand and tune in the most to my feelings about not having children. I remember the first time after my tubal pregnancy when he really comprehended that I couldn't have children. He looked *so* sad. My mother had kind of dismissed it and said I should be relieved, that kids can be a real pain. I knew she didn't mean it, because she's always loved being a mother. That was her way of trying to make me feel better.

"It was two or three years before I really talked to them about *my* feelings. They didn't say much; they're not really verbal people. But several months later, for Mother's Day, they sent me this beautiful Mother's Day card for a daughter. They said what a wonderful daughter I'd always been and how much they'd always loved me. It really choked me up. They didn't refer to my not being able to have children, but I knew they were thinking about it and trying to comfort me, telling me they care about my feelings. It means a lot."

Isabel too benefited from sharing her feelings with family members. Her parents chose not to respond verbally, but nonetheless they conveyed their love and concern through the card they sent.

STEP SIX

Using Available Resources

A wide array of resources exists beyond the circle of close friends and relatives, but you must be willing to use them. Some women believe that seeking outside help is a sign of inferiority or inadequacy. Others, overwhelmed by their depression and loss, withdraw and fail to consider alternative ways of handling their feelings. Do not let yourself fall into either trap. A wise person uses whatever resources are available.

RELIGION

Throughout the ages religion, or spirituality, a term many prefer, has been a source of inner strength and solace for people struggling with loss and disappointment. Religion can reaffirm life's meaning and order, even in the darkest of times, and it can bring perspective on the grand scheme of life by helping us see beyond our unique problems and situations.

Religion may not necessarily mean an organized church for you, but if you have not attended church services for years, you might visit different churches and see if one fits you. Along with other benefits, church membership often brings a supportive network into your life. However, if you know that organized religion is not what you want, explore other paths to a spiritual connection. Many people who have had negative experiences with organized religion lose touch with their own spirituality in the process of breaking away from a church. That does not have to happen, and I think it is unfortunate when it does. We all have a spiritual component that needs attention and nurturing; we are more than just physical, mental, and emotional beings.

Church is not the only place, and organized religion not the only way, that we can nurture our spirituality. We can also experience it in the secular realm as we go about our daily lives. Communing with nature inspires spiritual feelings in many people who experience a oneness with the world around them as they contemplate the beauty and order of the universe. I know a walk beside the ocean always comforts me. The ceaseless motion of the waves acts as a natural tranquilizer; it reminds me of the eternal nature of our universe and gives me a clearer perspective on my problems and disappointments. Planetarium shows also have a profound effect on me. For an hour or so, I lose myself in travels to distant stars and galaxies. Awed by the vastness and glory of the heavens, I return, when the show ends, to our tiny planet, which is but one dot among millions, to find I have a more realistic, a comforting appreciation of my relative importance in the universe. We cannot make these peaceful, spiritual moments happen, but we can welcome and treasure them when they occur. As is true with any kind of experience (meeting new people, learning about modern art), when our mind is open to its happening, our environment often produces the experience for us.

THERAPY

Therapy provides an opportunity for great healing and growth. Because of the one-dimensional nature of the therapeutic relationship, you do not need to take care of anyone but yourself, an unusual position for many women, who focus much of their time and energy on others. You can concentrate on your needs, your hurts, your life, in a nonjudgmental, secure environment. Because an objective, trained therapist participates in your therapy, you are supported through emotional upheavals, challenged to make new connections between events in your life, and encouraged to try new behavior.

Many people, especially those who have never tried it, discount the efficacy of therapy. Often, when a woman comes to see me because of marital problems, if she is able to persuade her reluctant mate to join us for a session, this is what I hear: "People have to solve their own problems. No one else can do it for them." While it is true that therapists have no magic, it is just as true that a professional can facilitate any endeavor (improving a golf game, planning for retirement, learning the right foods to eat after a heart attack). All of these situations, like the situations addressed in therapy, can be improved by a determined individual who does it on his or her own, but having a professional guide can help support and direct the process. Therapy is a shortcut to reaching your goals.

The more traumatic childlessness has been, the more likely it is that therapy will be beneficial. As you read previous steps in this book, you may have identified problems that indicate therapy would be helpful. In Step 1, acknowledging and experiencing the loss, did you feel that you are still too vulnerable, that you cannot yet open yourself to feeling the loss? In Step 2, understanding the loss, did you learn that your reasons for wanting a child were mainly hidden reasons, such as trying to compensate for a painful lack of good mothering in your own life? In Step 3, surviving the loss, did you realize you *do not* feel you have a right to be happy? In Step 4, letting go of blame, did you find that none of the exercises helped, that you are still caught up in endless blaming of yourself or others? In Step 5, talking to significant others, did you realize you have no one, no significant others, to whom you *can* talk? If so, perhaps you should consider therapy.

You may have to shop around to find a therapist who is right for you. Of course, you must choose someone with whom you feel comfortable, but you also need someone who will do more than hold your hand. You need a therapist who understands your feelings *and* challenges you to move on. While finding the right therapist may take time and effort, it is worth it. I have been on both sides of the therapeutic relationship, as a therapist as well as a client, and I know therapy can be a rich learning experience, a relationship that enriches both parties.

Many people who desire therapy never seek it because they fear it is too expensive. If you pay privately, it may well be, but many insurance policies will pay for a limited number of sessions. Nonprofit agencies such as Family Service, Catholic Charities, and Jewish Community Centers use a sliding-scale fee, so payment depends on your financial situation. Your local United Way should be able to suggest counseling agencies that you can afford. Many pastors, priests, and rabbis receive training in both religious and psychological counseling, and they offer services at no cost. If you live near a medical school or university that offers social work or psychology degrees, you may be able to see an intern at a reduced fee. If you want therapy, do not just assume you cannot afford it; check out the resources available in your area.

Role models

From the time we are children we pattern ourselves after people we respect. We may do this unconsciously, or we may consciously seek out role models. Many childless women search for and find examples of other childless women they admire, women who have created interesting, fulfilling lives.

Role models can provide inspiration. One woman was inspired by Katharine Hepburn. "I admire her tremendous spirit and dignity," she told me. "She has such *presence*. She didn't have children, and look at what an interesting, productive life she has had." Another woman mentioned Rosa Parks. "I respect her so much," she said. "I'm inspired when I think of the courage it took for her to refuse to give up her bus seat to a white man. Everyone has troubles, and when I face my troubles, I want to show the same quiet courage Rosa Parks showed."

Role models also help us feel less alone. Childless women often feel isolated, different from other women around them. If you feel there is no one who understands how you feel, reading about other women who have experienced a similar sadness will lessen your sense of isolation and loneliness.

OTHER CHILDLESS WOMEN

An aunt, an older colleague, or a neighbor or friend who is childless may be a resource, too. Consider asking them, "What helped you? How did you make your peace when you couldn't have children? What do you see as the benefits of childfree living?" Perhaps you can learn concrete coping skills that worked for them.

One woman felt better when an aunt who had worked up a family tree from the "old country" told her that often half of the eight or more children in a single family had no children. She concluded that her problem was probably related to family genes, and she felt less alone knowing others had had problems, too. Another woman took comfort from the fact that her older sister did not have children but was happy with her life.

Older childless women can also provide a longitudinal view. If you are in your twenties, thirties, or even forties, you might wonder how childlessness will affect you ten or twenty years from now. By asking women you know, you will learn about the different stages they have gone through and will probably find comfort in knowing you will not always feel the way you do now.

Groups

Women with infertility problems may have access to therapy groups sponsored by their doctors or clinics. Usually such groups have a therapist who acts as a facilitator; women who participated in such groups found them to be supportive and helpful. The national organization *Resolve,* which has local chapters scattered across the country, is also open to women with infertility problems. This group evolved from the shared pain of infertile couples and offers educational materials, peer counseling, and support groups. Although many of the group's members eventually have or adopt children, *Resolve* recognizes and supports the final decision of other members to remain childfree.

Self-help groups, which do not use a professional to facilitate interactions between group members, can also be beneficial. If you know of such a group for childless women, you may wish to join. Part IV of this book suggests ways to organize and start such a group yourself.

Retreats, Workshops, and Seminars

Many local colleges and churches offer growth-oriented programs in which the focus is not specifically on childlessness, but the programs may be helpful nonetheless. Workshops on loss are particularly relevant. Even though everyone's loss may be different—a loss due to body changes, like breast cancer, or the loss of a loved one due to death or divorce—the *experience and resolution* of loss are similar for everyone, which means members can relate to and learn from each other. Classes and workshops that focus on dreams provide a format for exploration of your deeper consciousness; they bring to awareness new possibilities in your life about which you are, literally, dreaming. Look for workshops that focus on identifying and pursuing new life goals. Such workshops help you to focus on attainable goals and to plan practical steps to reach them. Classes in meditation help you learn to find your quiet inner strength.

Books

If you like to read, if, like me, you are a woman who considers books an essential part of life, you might want to read the books listed in the bibliography. They are books I found helpful. If you cannot find them at a bookstore or library, ask your local librarian to arrange an interlibrary loan. A small fee may be charged, but almost any book can be located and forwarded to your local library.

The varied resources discussed above are in no way exhaustive, but they are readily available to almost everyone. If you find yourself going around in circles with your thoughts, your feelings, or your life, it is time to break out of your closed system. Most childless women *do* use available resources when they are ready to put the pain behind them and get on with the business of living; they choose those that fit their needs and personalities.

"Up from the Depths of Hell"

MARIA'S STORY

Maria grew up in El Paso, part of a large, disorganized, everyone-look-out-for-themselves family. She married at twenty-three. When she learned, at twenty-eight, that she could not have children because of infertility problems, she went into a deep depression. She got involved in a sexual affair that nearly destroyed her marriage, and she started drinking and almost killed herself in a car accident. Maria had been religious in her youth but had drifted away from her church.

"I've had bad times in my life, but when I had the accident and then my husband learned I'd been unfaithful, that was definitely the worst time in my life. I really wondered if I was going down for the last time, but I was saved by a loving God, who had other plans for me. My husband was offered a job in another state, and we decided to move and make a fresh start.

"We started going to church, and we were really lucky because the congregation we joined was warm and supportive. They adopted us; they let us know we were loved. The priest is very human, and he helped me see that God forgave me for all the awful things I'd done. My husband forgave me, too, and eventually I learned to forgive myself.

"I accept now that it's God's will whether or not we have children. Having children brings blessings and suffering, and not having children brings different blessings and different suffering. God gives each of us individual abilities and strengths, and when you don't have children, you just have to look harder to find these.

"Being close to God again brought a new meaning to my life. Now I accept it and all the blessings I have. My spiritual beliefs have been the most important factor in my healing. It's because I let God into my life that I've been able to bring myself up from the depths of hell, the hell I created. I can't tell you what it means to know there is a God who loves me, a God who looks after the universe. The spiritual aspect of this experience goes very deep."

Maria found her peace by returning to the organized religion of her youth. She was lucky to immediately find a congregation and priest that felt welcoming and comforting to her. Her religious beliefs have helped her forgive herself for things she wishes she had not done, and they provide her with a framework wherein her childlessness becomes acceptable.

"I Looked for Role Models"

SARAH'S STORY

Sarah, a thirty-eight-year-old woman who heads the consumer relations department of a national corporation, dreams of being an artist. In her free time she attends art classes. For six of the ten years since her divorce, she has been involved with a man who has children from a previous marriage. He is reluctant to marry again and does not want more children. Although she loves him, Sarah recently started to see other men because she would like to marry and have children if possible.

"I'm a great reader, and I looked for role models in women who have had successful and rewarding careers without children. I wondered how other women coped with this overwhelming need to have children, how they resolved it in terms of their own lives. I've found that women who have a creative career, artists and writers, have more to offer me than do women in the business world.

"The first to come to my attention was Georgia O'Keeffe. She made the achingly painful decision not to have children, and as a result all her creative energy was available for her art. Frida Kahlo, the wife of Diego Rivera, used her art to resolve her deep pain about being childless. Several of her paintings depict her fantasy of being a mother.

"Another role model for me is Gloria Steinem. In her book *Outrageous Acts and Everyday Rebellions* there is a section where she talks about being drawn to older people, which is the direction her maternal, nurturing instincts have always taken. I don't feel drawn to older people that way, but I do feel that I have a lot to contribute to adults my own age who need nurturing.

"I also found it helpful to talk to older childless women. I asked a good friend who's in her fifties how she felt about being childless at that age. She told me that she went through different stages at different times in her life, that it does get easier, which I found comforting."

Sarah found her salvation in a totally different way. She turned to books, where she found role models who showed how other women had dealt with their childlessness, role models who left no doubt in her mind that a childless woman could lead a full, creative, useful life.

STEP SEVEN

Rechanneling Mothering Energy

The need to nurture is often a powerful force for childless women. Although some women feel the need more intensely than others, most women experience tremendous frustration at one time or another because they have not expressed this potent bottled-up energy. To ensure survival of the human species, nature endowed us with this strong biological need, but the need is more than just physical; it is also psychological, social, and spiritual. We are dealing with a powerful force here, a force that demands expression and direction.

Like any driving need that motivates humankind—love, ambition, religion, sexual gratification, pride—the drive to mother can be a constructive or a destructive force. If you are immobilized by grief because you are childless, you already know the drive's destructive capabilities. Even when a woman has children, mothering energy can be negative. We all know mothers who smother their children, do everything for them, allow the children no independence, no life of their own. That is mothering energy gone awry. Since redirected energy can be either positive or negative as well, it must be channeled appropriately, and at the right time.

Timing

If, in the early stages of childlessness, when you first feel the loss, you fill your life with other activities as a way of avoiding your feelings, you are not really redirecting mothering energy; you are just denying your loss. A certain amount of grief work, of letting go, *must* take place first. Otherwise, the intention comes from the will and the mind and not from a resolved heart.

Other people, in well-meaning but misdirected attempts to comfort and help, often give advice that, on the surface, looks identical to this step. When I first told a social worker friend how much loss I felt at not having a child, she said, "I know, but there are lots of people around who need mothering. You can mother them." At that point I did not *want* to mother anyone or anything but my own child. The time we can hear such advice and act on it is *not* when we are first dealing with loss. The mourning and letting go must come first.

Overcompensating

Sometimes, in our first attempts to rechannel this energy, we overcompensate; we go to extremes in the opposite direction. Because we do not want to sit around and brood about not having children, we eagerly seek another focus for this energy; we throw ourselves into good causes with a frenzy that leaves us exhausted. One woman told me she had volunteered to be a teacher's assistant at her local school, a Big Sister to two girls, and on the board of two nonprofit agencies that offered children's services. She took on too much, wore herself out, and had to quit everything.

BROADENING OUR CONCEPT OF MOTHERING

The prevailing cultural attitude toward children, especially young children, is that they are the property of their biological or adoptive parents, an attitude that effectively shuts childless women out of the closed family circle. Many parents tend to think, or at least act, as though they *own* their children, and unfortunately our laws reflect and support this belief. That is one reason why physical and sexual abuse of children has been tolerated for so long. Parents had the right to treat their children as they saw fit. Only recently have children's rights begun to be recognized as legitimate, even when they conflict with parental rights.

This "ownership" attitude toward children results in small, isolated family units of parents and children—now it is often only one parent with children—who receive little support and help from anyone. The mobility of modern society results in many people living far away from their own parents or families of origin. There are not the grandmothers down the block, the sisters and aunts and cousins a telephone call away who will step in when help is needed. We lack the broad foundation of extended family that, until the last few generations, helped raise and nurture children. Oddly enough, in the same communities we have equally isolated childless women, men, and couples who play little significant part in the lives of families with children. They have no responsibilities and no rights toward these children.

Fortunately, not all people and cultures view the relationship between parents and children in such a restrictive way. Even before

I knew I would not have children, I was struck by Kahlil Gibran's *different* attitude about children. In his book *The Prophet* he says:

> Your children are not your children.
> They are the sons and daughters of Life's longing for itself.
> They come through you but not from you,
> And though they are with you yet they belong not to you.

In the book *Childlessness Transformed: Stories of Alternative Parenting,* Brooke Medicine Eagle speaks of "a beautiful and very functional tradition" among her Crow Indian people. She says, "*When a person has no children, then all the children are their children.* This means both all the children of that specific tribe, camp or clan as well as all the children of Earth, which includes every being and thing upon our Mother Earth."

How uplifting it would be for everyone if our culture made a significant mind shift on this issue. Imagine a society where children belong to us all, where all adults share responsibility for all children's well-being, where we all have a meaningful role to play. Such a society is idealistic, but for our own purposes we can adopt the concept that children belong to us all; we can decide *not* to be restricted by our culture. *We can decide to broaden our concept of mothering and free ourselves to find new ways to mother.*

When we do so, we are free to direct our untapped mothering love and nurturing energy where we feel it is most needed. We are not tied to just our own children. We can choose to mother all children (or adults or animals or the planet) in our lives with kindness and humor and love. We can pioneer new relationships, new structures. We can become part of extended, if surrogate, families. A single woman friend of mine recently became the West Coast grandmother for her friend's baby boy. Many women become "aunts" to their friend's children. Most of us know people with children—

neighbors, friends, colleagues, or relatives—who would be delighted to have other caring adults develop a significant relationship with the children, and in Step 8 we will talk more about the joys and the ways of including children in our lives.

HOW TO RECHANNEL MOTHERING ENERGY

1. *Deciding you want to.* The first step, not surprisingly, is deciding if you *need and want* to find a new focus for your untapped energy. Not all of you will feel this need; you may have already compensated for not having children and be content. But if you *do* feel unsatisfied, if you feel as though something significant is missing in your life, you need to pursue this step. If you are not certain, ask yourself the following questions:

- Do you feel you have parts of yourself you want to share but no one with whom you can share them?
- Have you considered but not acted on a desire to become involved with projects or causes outside yourself?
- When you picture yourself making changes and getting involved with children or other activities, do you feel excited? Do you feel more positive about yourself?

2. *Choosing a focus.* When we think of rechanneling our mothering energy, the most obvious choice is other children, and certainly there are many children who need nurturing, many ways we can become involved with children. Pediatric nurseries in hospitals often need volunteers to hold and comfort premature babies, who spend weeks or months institutionalized. Big Sister organizations match adult volunteers with girls who need more attention and stimulation

than their own families or environments can provide. Or you might enjoy leading a nature walk for children or reading stories to children at a local bookstore or library. There are many options.

But focusing on children is not the only possibility. Many women find great satisfaction in nurturing adults, sometimes frail older adults who need supportive services so they can stay in their own homes, or older adults who live in nursing homes. If this appeals to you, either volunteer through an organized program or develop a caring relationship with an older adult you know. Take the individual to a concert, to a ball game, or for a ride; run errands to the bank or post office; or simply visit, often the greatest gift of all.

Other women turn naturally to animals, either as pets or by becoming involved in broader causes such as marine mammal protection or working to save endangered species. Increasingly, many embrace the concept of mothering planet earth in an attempt to counter the pollution, exploitation, and nuclear destruction that threaten the planet. Other women prefer to direct their energies toward the creative arts or private enterprises.

3. *Challenging yourself.* Because women have traditionally been so focused on relationships and taking care of others, few have ever *really* tapped the depth and breadth of their intellectual, physical, or creative abilities. If they think about it at all, they *would* like to do more with their lives, but they hold back. The reasons why are legion. Because they have never been encouraged to reach for the stars, they hardly dare dream at all. They fear that if they break the old mold, they will irreparably damage significant relationships in their lives; they fear failure; they worry what others will say if they embark on some new adventure; they do not know just what it is they want to do. If this sounds like you, I highly recommend the book *Wishcraft: How to Get What You Really Want,* by Barbara Sher with Annie Gottlieb. It is a concrete, step-by-step guide to identifying and getting what you want.

You can also use what you learned about yourself in Step 2, understanding the loss. Go back to the notes you made then and examine once again your reasons for wanting a child. Identify once more the hardest part for you of being childless. Let yourself feel again the unmet needs of your inner child. Herein will lie clues to how you can best rechannel your mothering energy so that you bring into your life that which you hoped to experience through mothering.

When we dreamed of having children, we wanted to bring our finest qualities, our purest love to mothering. We wanted to be the best we could be as mothers. Just because we do not have children is no reason to neglect those finest qualities, that purest love, that striving to be the best that we can be.

"Don't Waste It"

SALLY'S STORY

When Sally married, she was thirty-seven, and her husband was forty-eight. They hoped to have children and tried for several years before undergoing infertility studies. Her husband had a low sperm count that could not be corrected, and neither of them wanted to adopt because of their ages. Sally and her husband own and operate a dry-cleaning business.

"I think it's so important that childless women take their nurturing energy and don't waste it. We have to use it positively in other ways. When a woman has a child, her energy is focused, but because our energy doesn't have a focal point, it's chaotic, just flinging around wondering where the hell to go. It's no good to just stuff it in a pocket, because it can get out of hand. It can become a monster that ruins your life. We have to focus it as best we can.

"Women have to be careful, though, that they don't mishandle this energy. At first, when I was trying to accept that I would never have a child, I went overboard trying to use my mothering energy. I became a do-gooder. I tried to solve all the world's problems. Show me a wrong, and I tried to right it. I was ready to join any crusade, whatever the cause. I was trying to be a supermom to the whole world, and I wore myself out. Now I know how to moderate it.

"Two years ago I won a highly competitive race for the local hospital board. Staff morale was low, and the administration was ineffective. We had to go in and completely reorganize the hospital. I'm developing new skills, which excites me. I see that I'm creating a role for myself that includes being a nurturer. The hospital needed people who could help to bring about a sense of self-esteem for everyone in the system, and I'm finding that I can do this, in addition to more traditional board functions. Could only a woman with a lot of extra love to give do this? I don't know. But I've found a place to use what I have, and it feels good."

Childless women are obviously not the only people who involve themselves in civic causes or give of themselves outside their own circle of family and friends, but doing so has a special meaning for them. It is a way to rechannel the mothering energy that otherwise would go untapped.

"I Have as Many Children as I Choose to Have"

ALICE'S STORY

Alice is the oldest of four children. She describes herself as "a former hippie, whatever that means." Her unconventional life-style caused conflict between her and her parents when she was younger, and she moved to California from her home in Michigan to get away from the family problems. She is now fifty-four, loves to garden, works in a health food store, and devotes her free time to environmental causes.

"Since my twenties I've had serious political doubts about having children. I wasn't sure it was going to be such a wonderful world to grow up in. I also distrusted many of my motives for wanting a child, so I decided to wait until I was truly ready. When I was thirty-six I felt ready, and the man I was with at the time wanted children too. My first pregnancy ended in a miscarriage after five months, and the second one was a tubal pregnancy that left me incapable of having children. I was disappointed, but I don't worship childbearing, and I wasn't going to make it my religion, so I accepted the inevitable. It's not been the tragedy of my life.

"I have come to know that I don't have to have 'my own' children to feel fulfilled or complete. That ownership fantasy is a BS creation of the patriarchy. I really feel that I am *not* a woman without a child, because I have as many children as I choose to have by seeing all children as my own. Whether I'm talking to a child in a shopping cart at the checkout line or tending a neighbor's child for an afternoon, these children are mine for that time, and I treat them as such. Why do we have kids but to use them as a vehicle to share the love within us? I think there should be childless women in every community. Our love is more free floating. We pick up a lot of the slack in the world.

"I highly recommend therapy or counseling to any woman who isn't getting what she wants from her life. The time is over when women have to settle for less than they really want. There are so many options today."

Alice took her childlessness in stride. She has many other interests, many other projects. What I find most impressive about Alice's story is that when she has contact with a child, even if it is only in the checkout line at a grocery store, that child is hers for the moment. As a result, Alice feels she is *not* a woman without a child; she has as many children as she chooses to have by seeing all children as her own.

Including Children in Your Life

If you approach this step with a jaundiced eye because you think I will try to persuade you that including children in your life will compensate for not having children of your own, you can relax. One assumption underlies everything I say: *there is no substitute for having children of your own.*

Some childless women choose, deliberately or unconsciously, *not* to be involved with children because they know that involving themselves with a godchild or stepchildren, caring for nieces and nephews, being a Big Sister, or volunteering at a school or at a pediatric ward will not be the same as having children of their own. And they are right. But these different activities are not *meant* to be the same as being a mother; they are not even meant to be substitutes. They are entirely different experiences. *Do not expect alternative ways of being with children to compensate for being childless; if you do, you will set yourself up for disappointment.*

That said, there is no reason—just because you do not have children of your own—why you should deprive yourself of the fun and pleasure of being with children. I am admittedly enthusiastic about this step; my life has been greatly enriched by the children who are a part of it.

Choosing Roles

The role of mother is in many ways a highly proscribed one having to do with the activities of daily living. Mothers are expected to socialize their children, which means tremendous amounts of time and energy must be directed at what children should and should not do. We all know mothers' familiar litanies. Eat your vegetables! Clean up your room! Don't hit your little sister! Every mother I know intended, when her first baby was born, to focus on the positive, to limit the number of "nos!" and "don'ts!" that the child heard. Yet soon these same mothers hear themselves saying the very words they vowed to avoid (and often saying them in the same tone of voice their mothers used). It goes with the territory of being a mother. One advantage of not being a mother, then, is that your relationship with a child need not be so defined and constrained. It is not your job to socialize the child.

You have much more flexibility and freedom to choose the role you want to play. One woman saw herself as playing an Auntie Mame role. If you remember Rosalind Russell in the movie *Auntie Mame,* you will understand immediately that this woman had no wish to socialize her nieces and nephews. She wanted to be outrageous with them. She wanted to show them the delights of an unconventional life beyond the constraints of social mores.

Another woman became the trusted adult confidante of her friend's teenage children. She knew far more than the parents did of what really went on in the teenagers' lives, and she loved being the wise adviser. Other women enjoy being *the* adult who introduces a child to music or art or sports, *the* adult who sees a child's interests and talents and helps cultivate them. The bond of their shared interests can last a lifetime.

Whether you already have children in your life or are considering making room for them, think about the role(s) you would really enjoy playing. What unique part of yourself had you hoped to share with your children? What part of yourself do you value the most? Is there a neglected part of yourself just waiting to blossom? The answers to these questions will give you insight into the kind of relationships *you* would most enjoy having with children.

CHOOSING ACTIVITIES

To get the most out of your relationship with children, plan special activities that you will enjoy, too. Think back and remember the outings and games and projects that you enjoyed as a child—and just might enjoy again. Did you like to play in the sandbox with a pail and shovel? Was finger painting a favorite activity? Did you like camping trips complete with tents, bonfires at night, and roasting hot dogs and marshmallows? How long since you have seen a children's movie?

Or think back and remember the things you always wanted to do but did not do as a child, for whatever reason. Did you always want to collect seashells or stamps? Learn to ice-skate or ride horseback? Climb trees, build model airplanes, sew clothes for a favorite doll? Tell ghost stories late at night? Contact with children gives us a reason to do things we would not ordinarily do; it gives us an excuse to let our inner child out to play. One woman, who was an only child, told me she always wished she had lots of brothers and sisters to play with as a child. "I think that carried over into my adulthood," she said. "I'm still looking for kids to play with."

POTENTIAL PITFALLS

Problems can also arise, of course, when you open your heart and your life to children. If you know in advance what the potential problems are, you are in a better position to cope with them if they do arise.

The greatest danger (dangerous because it can be so hurtful) is that you lose or are denied contact with the children who are important to you. Sometimes life events—a move out of state, a dwindling friendship with the child's family, a single parent's remarriage—will result in changes that gradually bring less contact. Sometimes, though, the break is more traumatic. Since you serve, if you will, at the pleasure of the parents, you are subject to their whims and caprices. If they wish, they can stop your contact with the child at any time, for any reason. A number of women I interviewed had had very painful experiences along these lines.

Mary, for example, lived with a man for four years and told me that his two children, who spent alternate weekends and many holidays with them, were as important to her as her lover. She loved the children, and they loved her. When the children's father decided to leave the relationship, she lost not only the man she loved but his children as well. The children's mother did not want Mary to continue to see the children, and she had no entree, no "legitimate" claim to do so. She never saw them again.

Another woman, Missy, married a widower who had adult children. His only son lived near them and was active with his father in the family business. When the son and his wife had their first child, a boy, Missy was welcomed as the paternal grandmother. All went well for six years, until business-related problems created a bitter rift between her husband and his son. Missy's close, loving relationship with the boy suffered as a result.

Being cut off from a child you love is not unique to childless women, of course. When there is a divorce or when one parent dies, grandparents, aunts, and uncles often find themselves unable to effectively maintain contact with a child to whom they were once close. Any loving relationship can go astray. This brings to mind the age-old question: is it better to love and lose than never to have loved at all? Reworded for purposes of this discussion, is it better to have children in your life (with all the joy and fun and love such contact brings) and lose those children, or is it better never to have had the contact at all? Each woman must answer for herself, of course. I believe that life-affirming people have always answered yes to love, yes to relationships, even though there are risks. For most of us, life's greatest meaning and pleasure come from the loving relationships we have with other people. To gain, we must risk.

Another less significant but nonetheless annoying problem that arises is hearing from a child's parents, "What do *you* know? You don't have children!" This response is usually given when you offer opinions or observations the parents do not want to hear. You may in fact *know* some very important things about the child, whether you have children or not. However, the child's parents find it easier to dismiss your opinion—because you are not a mother—than to evaluate what you have to say.

Again, this is not unlike interactions that take place in other relationships. We all weigh whether or not to level with a friend about her exploitive boyfriend or tell a colleague we think she has an alcohol problem. Any opinions can be rebuffed, but when the opinion is rejected because we are not mothers, our greater vulnerability comes into play. If you think the parents might not welcome your opinion about the child and her needs, proceed cautiously. If you feel you must speak up regardless, try to communicate in a noncritical, nonthreatening manner.

Another potential pitfall you should prepare for is the transition time when you return a child to her parents. You may have had a marvelous time with the child; you both have laughed and played and enjoyed each other's company. You return triumphant; you *know,* you *feel,* how much you mean to the child. But be prepared—when the child sees home and mother and siblings and friends, you are usually forgotten. The child rushes away from you without a backward glance. The younger the child, the truer this is. The first time or two this happens, you may feel as though you have been hit in the stomach with a sledgehammer, as though a door has been slammed in your face. Learn to disengage and distance as transition time approaches. We all learn to do this with other transitions, for example, on Sunday night, when we let go of the weekend and start to think of work the next day, or when vacations or visits are winding down.

Not all partings are difficult, of course. You may feel gratified when you see how reluctant the child is to say good-bye, how eager he is to know when he will see you next. And many, many childless women report (with great amusement) how relieved they are to return children to their rightful parents. After a day or even a few hours with a child, many women are worn out; they are the ones who are eager to say good-bye.

Bask in Being Special

If you invest in children, it will not be long before you see that you *are* important to them. It may be the smile on a toddler's face when he sees you, or the excited cry at the airport, "Aunt Kathie, Aunt Kathie," when you fly in for Thanksgiving. It may be a teenage neighbor's shy suggestion that maybe she could come over sometime and talk to you about her boyfriend. Whatever it is, when you know you are special, let yourself enjoy it. Bask in it.

Many women I interviewed acted as though they felt compelled to discount their importance to a child. They would describe with animation and obvious pleasure a trip to Disneyland with nieces or the closeness that developed when they tended a friend's child every day after school or the special relationship they had with children they taught. And then they stopped themselves, put a cap on their excitement, as though some judgment had taken place inside their heads. "Of course I'm only an aunt [or only a teacher or only a neighbor], not a mother," they would say, the underlying assumption obviously being that mothers matter, aunts (and teachers and neighbors) do not. Nonsense! Children need many different adults in their lives. You may well be giving a child something he or she gets from no one else.

Being a favorite aunt is a very special position, one that can provide rich, loving, enduring relationships that last a lifetime. The same is true for stepmothers, godmothers, neighbors, teachers, nurses, doctors, and librarians. Whatever role you play, if you care about the child and the child cares about you, cherish the relationship; do not discount it to yourself or others because you are not the child's mother.

FOCUS ON THE MOMENT

If you decide to involve yourself with children, learn to focus on the moment, to live in the present. Soak up the laughter, the fun, the spontaneity. Do this for two reasons. The first reason is because you will experience life more fully and your pleasure will increase. The present, the *now,* is where we actually live our lives; the past is behind us, the future before us. If you develop the art of focusing your attention on the moment, you will feel more alive; your enjoyment of life will increase.

A second reason to do so is that you will be better able to cope when your heart is suddenly pierced by the longing for a child of your own. For you *will* have times—whether you are holding a toddler on your lap, enjoying the body contact, the warmth, looking down at the angelic face; or romping on the beach with a nephew, splashing in the waves; or having a philosophical discussion with a like-minded teenager—when you suddenly feel a great sadness, an emptiness. "If only I had had a child," you will think. When it happens, do not deny the feeling, just refocus on the present. The child you wanted to have is beyond your reach, but here, now, in the present you are with a child, you are experiencing a moment that will never come again. Cherish it.

"Enjoy It for What It Is"

LOIS'S STORY

Lois's early childhood was chaotic because her mother was schizophrenic and spent long periods in a state mental hospital. Each time her mother was hospitalized, Lois was sent to live with a different relative. Because of her early experiences, she was ambivalent about being a mother herself. She worries about her ability to bond with and care for a child.

"My therapist asked me once, 'Does it have to be all or nothing? Isn't there something in between?' I thought about that. For several years I'd wondered what it would be like to volunteer as a Big Sister. I couldn't do it until last year, but I decided it might be okay, as long as I didn't try and make that the substitute for having children.

"The Little Sister they assigned to me is ten. I do things with her that I would have liked to do with my own child. I take her to movies; I ask about school. It's been good for me to get involved with her. It's helped me to get out of myself.

"I make a date to go with her once a week, and often when the time comes, I don't want to go. It's funny how I resist it. But I know enough now *not* to give in to the resistance. I *make* myself go, and then I'm glad I did. Now that she's used to me, she's open and very affectionate. When I open my heart up a little bit to receive some of that affection, I do feel better. I realize it's helped me as much as it's helped her. I think more and more the solution for me is to just do the concrete, practical actions that I know make me feel better, like being with her even when I don't feel like it.

"When I left my Little Sister in the beginning, I would be jealous of her mother, and I would feel sort of sorry for myself. I'd think, 'This doesn't take the place of having a child myself.' But then I realized that this is something different, and I can enjoy it for what it is.

"My very closest friend is expecting soon, and she wants me to be actively involved with the baby. I get scared when I think about risking closeness and involvement. What if they move away? In the past I would have run away. I *have* run away from other friends with kids, but that doesn't seem to be the answer, to insulate yourself. This time I'm going to go with it anyway and get involved. I'm going to take the risk."

Lois was ambivalent about including children in her life, and she first tested the waters by being a Big Sister. She found that to be an acceptable, enjoyable experience. Now she is ready to risk greater closeness and involvement with her friend's baby. I would predict that that relationship will bring even greater pleasure.

"A Feeling of Being a Mother"

NORENE'S STORY

Norene would have liked to have children, but when the years went by and she did not marry, she easily accepted her childlessness. She liked her career as a real-estate broker, had many friends, and enjoyed being an aunt to her eight nieces and nephews. When, at forty-five, she met the man who was to become her husband, she was delighted that he had a daughter.

"I've found tremendous satisfaction in being a stepmother. Leslie, my stepdaughter, is going to be twenty-five this month, and I've helped raise her from the time she was ten. She and I became very close when her father and I were seeing each other, but there was a bit of an adjustment after the marriage. She was afraid I'd try to replace her mother, which she didn't want. I knew enough not to do that, and soon our relationship was very, very good.

"Now that Leslie is grown up and married and on her own, I mother her more than I did when she was younger. I guess we had to grow into the relationship. She's expecting a baby now, and I'm very excited. We go shopping together for baby clothes, and she wants me to help her once the baby is born. I feel like I'll be a full-fledged grandmother, because I'll be there from the beginning, not entering in the middle of the act like you do with stepchildren. The baby will always know me as his or her grandmother.

"I've been lucky. Not all childless women have the chance to mother someone else's children. I'm not suggesting that having stepchildren is an instant solution to childlessness. It's definitely not the same as having your own baby, but it can be wonderful. Leslie has really given me a feeling of being a mother."

Many childless women who are stepmothers develop close relationships with their stepchildren. Sometimes the relationship has overtones of mothering; often it partakes more of friendship. Leslie will soon know the joys of being a grandmother. She and I and other childless women who get to be grandmothers are blessed indeed.

STEP NINE

Maximizing the Advantages of Childfree Living

When we humans invest emotionally in a decision, a plan, an idea, we tend to close our minds to sound, persuasive arguments that support other opinions. Often the issue in question is not one of right or wrong, but rather a question of the relative merits of two different things. Still we stubbornly refuse to acknowledge the positive aspects of the side the other person champions. If you have ever participated in or overheard a discussion about whether walking or running is better for your health, whether Paris or London offers the visitor more pleasures, whether it is preferable to start your own business or work for others, you know what I mean. Both alternatives in the examples have merit; both have drawbacks.

And so it is with childlessness. Because we feel so strongly what we *have lost* by being childless, we are reluctant to admit, even to ourselves, that there *are* advantages to our situation. But advantages there definitely are. The fact that the advantages *may not* outweigh the losses for you does not invalidate their existence.

Many childless women have times when they are glad they do not have children. That does not mean they would not still choose to *have had* children if their lives had been different. It does mean that in the moment, they see and appreciate the advantages of being childfree. Keep an open mind. You too may eventually have times when you feel that way. Be honest with yourself if you do. You do not have to feel guilty.

CHILDLESS? OR CHILDFREE?

A world of difference lies between the two words *childless* and *childfree*. The difference is one of attitude, but then attitude always *does* make a difference. Although you might like to will or force this change in perspective within yourself, you cannot. The ability to appreciate the advantages of a childfree life comes with resolution. If you try too early in the resolution process to adopt an attitude of, "Oh, well, I really don't mind not having children because now I can go out whenever I want and travel wherever I choose," you run the risk of rationalizing. Instead of dealing with your loss, you will be denying it and trying to avoid your feelings.

In the early stages of dealing with their childlessness, some women cannot even begin to imagine that the time will come when they think of themselves as childfree instead of childless. One woman was told by her uncle, "Some women are denied motherhood; others are relieved of it. It all depends on your perspective." At that time she was still dealing with the trauma of being childless, but his words stuck in her mind, and every now and then they would pop up unexpectedly, reminding her that there was another way to look at her situation. I had a similar experience. Some time during the years I was being treated for infertility, I heard the writer Alice Walker speak. During her talk she referred to something her mother had said about childless women, something to the effect of, "If the good Lord gives you that freedom, then enjoy it." At that point in my life being childless did not feel like freedom, but the words stayed with me, and now I know what she meant.

TIME

Time is a finite and highly democratic resource. We all, rich and poor alike, get twenty-four hours each day, no more, no less, to use as we see fit. We all spend chunks of time from our allotted hours doing chores we would rather not do: working, commuting, cleaning, ironing, cooking, standing in line, chauffeuring others. Obviously, the more demands on our time for practical, daily chores, the less time we have available for the activities we prefer. Of necessity, women with children spend more time doing all those things because, in addition to themselves, they are responsible for dependent children who need those services too; they may also be responsible for earning the money that helps support a family. Women without children have the advantage of having more time to use as they choose.

FINANCIAL RESOURCES

Most of us have limited financial resources. We must pick and choose how best to allocate the money we have. Rightly or wrongly, the salaries we earn take no account of a woman's economic need and the size of her family. Women with children are paid no more than are women without children, so the former must spread their limited resources more thinly. Childless women may have to make choices, such as whether to get the car fixed or get new carpeting, but we do not have to also factor in whether to buy Janie's new shoes or get our hair cut, whether to get braces for Tommy's teeth or go on vacation. We do not have to sacrifice our needs and wants because of children. When we look ahead to our retirement years, we can more readily invest and plan for our future, since we do not have the financial burden of college tuition to pay, perhaps for a decade or longer, in the case of families with several children.

ENERGY

The older we get, the more it seems that energy has its limits, too. This energy factor played a significant part in my resolution, because the time came when I felt too old to be a mother. After tending a baby for an evening or young children for a day, I realized, "I'm too old to start as a mother now! *My time has come and gone.*" Knowing that I would not choose to have a baby then, even if I had the choice, brought tremendous relief. This may not apply to some high-energy people who do not slow down, but as they grow older, most women appreciate being able to lie back with a good book or postpone cooking dinner when they are tired. Most mothers I know are tired much of the time, for obvious reasons. Those of us without children have far fewer demands on our energy.

RELATIONSHIPS WITH OTHER ADULTS

Women who have a significant partner in their lives have more time and energy to spend with that person. It is easier for couples without children to be more intimate, and I do not mean just sexually, although that is true as well. My husband and I had a foreign student live with us for a year. We thoroughly enjoyed the experience, and yet we felt like honeymooners when we were alone again.

Having children can create problems for a relationship. Many couples strongly disagree about the "right way" to raise children; usually when this is the case, the differences take their toll on the couple's relationship. From my family therapy experience, I know it is possible for one parent to form an alliance with one or more children against the other parent, effectively shutting that parent out of the family circle. Or a parent who feels closer to a child than to the spouse turns to that child for the emotional warmth and intimacy that rightfully belong in the marital relationship. Both configurations wreak havoc in a relationship.

When a woman has children, relationships with other adults—parents, siblings, and friends—must also conform to children's needs and schedules. Scheduled get-togethers with friends who are mothers often have to be canceled because a child is sick or the babysitter cannot make it. I know when my two sisters used to have, and my nieces now do have, lots of children vying for attention while we talk, it is impossible to have the kind of warm, sharing conversations we have when the children are not present. Those of us who do not have children are able to devote our full attention to these significant relationships.

FREEDOM AND FLEXIBILITY

A life without children lends itself more readily to spontaneity. Women with children are more constricted, more tied to routine. Whether it is deciding on a moment's notice to go out for dinner or take off for the weekend, we can choose to do so if we wish. If we find ourselves in work situations we do not like, we can more easily contemplate changes because we do not have the responsibility of providing food and shelter for others who cannot provide for themselves. This sense of being in control of one's life, of being able to make choices and changes as we like, is an important factor in an individual's perceived quality of life. No one likes to feel trapped.

OPPORTUNITY FOR SELF-DEVELOPMENT

Of all the advantages identified by the women I talked to, this one, the opportunity for self-development, was mentioned with the most heartfelt fervor. Mothers spend their best energy caring for others; they live their lives tending to others' growth and well-being, often at their own expense. Childless women know it is a special gift to have the time and space for their own development. Learning about oneself, growing and developing, bring tremendous satisfaction. Women tend to become more contemplative as they mature; they examine the twists and turns, the complexities and challenges, of their lives as they try to puzzle out how they got from where they started to where they are. They try to make sense of all that has happened to them. Childless women usually have more time and energy for this process. In Step 10, embracing the quest for feminine wholeness, we explore this advantage in depth.

SPARED HEARTACHES

Having children brings many joys *and* many heartaches. We may have missed the joys, but we *were* spared the heartaches. We are all acquainted with women who have known great sorrow because of their children's problems. Women who have developmentally disabled children say it is a heartache that never ends. The death of a child through illness, accident, or malice is devastating. Even when an adult child dies, parents often feel an irrational guilt, because they feel, given life's natural order, *they* should have been the ones to die first. Being a mother to an individual who gets involved with drugs, alcohol, or crime is a nightmare all its own. Mothers whose children turn against them for whatever reason are subjected to years of antagonism and being blamed; or, if the children distance themselves and break away completely, the mother is left alone and bereft. Parents' hearts ache, too, when their adult children go through divorces or when they can only stand by and watch helplessly as their children drift aimlessly and unsatisfactorily through life. Childless women are spared all this and more.

Learning to value what we have is an essential ingredient in the art of being happy. No one, at least no one I know, gets everything they want in life. But we can learn to appreciate and maximize the good things we do have.

"More Time to Find Myself"

LAVERNE'S STORY

We heard from LaVerne in Step 2 when she talked about wanting children for all the wrong reasons. LaVerne is a licensed vocational nurse and a recovering alcoholic who has been sober for nine years.

"There have been times I've been glad that I didn't have children, when my life was not stable because of my drinking problem, and recently when I went through a divorce. Then, too, I look at my sister's problems with her children—drugs, incompatibility, health problems—and I'm thankful I don't have to cope with that. A friend of mine recently lost a child, and I thought, 'At least I don't ever have to face the heartbreak of losing a child.'

"Another thing, I don't have to watch my children confront me with all the things I did wrong in raising them, nor do I have to regret in my own mind the mistakes I made. I think that must be one of the most difficult things a mother has to face.

"I know I've had more time to find myself—which I've needed. I spent my whole childhood and early adulthood living my mother's hopes and dreams, so it's taken me longer to come to terms with myself. One spinoff for other people is that I've given all my mothering to my patients. Even now I can lose myself in providing and planning and taking care of my patients' needs. I freely gave my mothering away; I mothered everyone coming down the pike. And it was very, very satisfying. Giving is the essence of my being. It gives me credibility for who I am."

Acknowledging the advantages of a childfree life does not mean an individual thinks she has a better life than women who are mothers. It means women are able to see the difference in the two life-styles and appreciate the pluses of *both*.

"I Have Seen Wonderful Sights"

EMILY'S STORY

Emily has always been interested in helping others. In her twenties she was a Peace Corps volunteer in Africa, and on her return to the States worked for several years helping an inner-city church set up a preschool. She is now forty-nine and has been married for six years. She plays the cello and enjoys sailing. She loves her work with young children in the preschool she runs.

"Although I've never been glad to be childless, I do know the compensations have been tremendous. It has allowed me to be more self-centered, because time and money and emotion, among other things, were not being spread among many people. I've been primarily responsible for myself, and thus I've been able to give more time to self-growth and self-discovery.

"I have greater independence and greater affluence. I'm free to do whatever I want without worrying about a babysitter or taking the children along. I know I'd have had to give up a lot of my freedom and mobility. I couldn't have traveled as I've done. And I know my life would be very different energywise if I had children; my time and energy would have to be reprogrammed. Now I have time for all the things I love, especially my music and backpacking trips. I'm blessed because my career allows me to be with children during the day, but I'm also able to maintain my life without children away from work.

"I have lived a very full life. I have lived in the Australian bush and in Africa. I have had many different kinds of jobs and have a great many friends, and much more adventure than perhaps the average person does. I have seen wonderful sights and felt wonderful new feelings that perhaps would not have been mine were I tied to life with a child."

Not only did Emily find ways to productively rechannel her mothering energy, she did it in a manner that allowed her to have wonderful adventures along the way. She used the greater affluence and independence of her childfree life for self-growth and self-discovery. She took advantage of childfree living.

S T E P T E N

Embracing the Quest for Feminine Wholeness

Childlessness has disrupted most of our lives at one time or another. It has forced us to confront our unmet needs, our heart's longings, and our exposed vulnerabilities. We have experienced a lack of harmony in our lives, either within ourselves or in our external world with surroundings and people and situations. Childlessness has left us feeling *not whole*.

Most people search for meaning in life, especially in times of crisis, and childless women's search for meaning is often inextricably linked to their childlessness. Disappointments and tragedies challenge our assumptions; they challenge our often unexamined beliefs and values. Difficult as crises are, they *do* set the stage for change. With the status quo in flux, our defenses are weakened, and we have less resistance to making psychological and behavioral changes. In this sense, childlessness presents an opportunity for personal growth.

Embracing the quest for feminine wholeness means embarking on an inward spiritual journey whereby we learn to know ourselves, learn to value ourselves. It means reaching deep within ourselves to discover previously untapped strength and wisdom, which we then use to create a fulfilling life without children. It means feeling whole again.

WHY WE DO NOT FEEL WHOLE

Who am I beyond the roles I play? is a question that troubles many women. To some degree, people define themselves, and are defined by others, according to the roles they play in society, roles that describe both the tasks they perform and their relationships with others, especially members of their own family. Women have been, and continue to be, defined rather rigidly by their relationships within the family: daughters, wives, mothers, and grandmothers are the primary ways women have been identified for generations. Only recently have we also been known as corporate executives, writers, stockbrokers, policewomen, and mechanics.

This is part of the reason why childlessness distresses us so much. Being a mother has been one of the two *most important* roles adult women have been expected to play: wife and mother. When women *with children* ask,"Who am I?"—and they do ask, because they do not define themselves exclusively as mothers—they can and do answer, "Well, I'm a mother, for one thing." The role of mother constitutes an important if partial answer to the question. When childless women ask, "Who am I?" they cannot fall back on the role of mother. They face a void.

At some deep level we feel that as women we are *supposed* to be able to have children. If we cannot or do not, then we often question our worth. The assumption that a woman who has a child is worth more than a woman who does not is obviously fallacious, if not downright silly, when carried to its logical conclusion: if we truly believe a woman who has a child has more value than a childless woman, then it follows logically that a woman with two children is worth more than a woman with one child, and a woman with six children is very valuable indeed, an obviously senseless argument. So even though society's definition of adult women as mothers is deeply cemented into our psyches, we can and should reexamine it. We need not accept it at face value. One of the challenges of resolution is seeing that being a woman is many different things; motherhood is just one possibility. When we accept that our value as a human being is not tied to having children, we give ourselves permission to be childless.

This question of identity manifests itself on a grander scale as well. We not only have difficulty knowing who we are as individuals; we also have trouble identifying our pure, innate feminine spirit. Masculine influence permeates everything from politics to architecture; it dominates every aspect of the world as we know it. No one knows what form education or government or business systems would take if they evolved from a feminine perspective. Because the female *spirit* differs from the dominant male spirit, we are at a disadvantage when we seek to identify feminine wholeness. We have few guidelines other than culturally prescribed ones, and they tell us what men believe and think is feminine. Women who consciously seek to discover and examine the pure female spirit face the uncertainty and exhilaration of a new frontier.

As women we have been socialized to take care of others at our own expense. We know more about the needs and wants of children, husbands, and parents than we know about our own needs and wants. Often we show more kindness and sensitivity to others than we do to ourselves. Most of us *do* enjoy nurturing those we love, but if we do not keep a healthy balance, our own identity can be swallowed up in an eager rush to please and nurture others. We can *lose* ourselves.

We may also feel less than whole because of our unique experiences. Many of us still feel wounds from the past. The wounding may have occurred in early childhood or adolescence. We may have been disappointed in love, or we may feel we have never had the opportunity to use our intelligence and abilities in ways we would like. We may feel that adult life is, after all, often disappointing. When we carry these hurts within us, we feel fragmented and torn apart.

EMPOWERING OURSELVES, AFFIRMING OURSELVES

Although there are notable exceptions, women as a whole do not, with any degree of comfort, think of themselves as powerful people. We tend to give our personal power away; we tend to turn it over to others. By personal power I mean the right and ability to decide what is right for us, the right and ability to say what we have to say, the right and ability to live our lives as we wish to live them.

Our early conditioning impedes us when we try to take control of our lives and develop our inner strength and self-reliance. We were taught to be nice and sweet and agreeable, and thus we find it hard to be outspoken, assertive, and decisive. We were sensitized never to act in ways that would threaten the egos of men who are important in our lives, and so, even as we long for self-direction, we have trouble speaking up for ourselves, trouble standing firm when we need to. It is no wonder that women so often feel powerless.

Thus another challenge of resolution is learning to affirm our own importance and to take ourselves seriously. We need to see that our own thoughts and feelings and desires are no less important than anyone else's. We need to rely on self-affirmation instead of relying on external affirmation. We need to incorporate into our everyday lives new behaviors that reflect our belief in our own importance. When we do, we reclaim our own power.

VISUALIZATION AND AFFIRMATION EXERCISES

Visualization and affirmation exercises are helpful ways to make the transition.

If you want to try visualization, find a time when you will not be disturbed or feel rushed. Read through the exercise first; then get comfortable, close your eyes, and relax.

Picture yourself in situations that mirror your actual life.

Visualize yourself as you want to be.

Imagine yourself acting and feeling as you would like to act and feel.

You are the artist; in your mind's eye create the *you* you want to be.

Refine the image. Run through it again.

Change anything you want to change until you are satisfied.

Now broaden the picture beyond the life you have today. Visualize changes you would like.

Would you continue to live where you do, or would you move?

Would you continue to do the same work, or would you try something different?

How much time would you spend with other people?

How much time would you spend with yourself?

Would you like to form new relationships?

What changes would you make in existing relationships?

Design the ideal world for you.

You will need to practice this visualization exercise on a regular basis. Before we can make something happen, we first need to know what it is we want. When we visualize ourselves as we want to be, when we picture the life we want to lead, we give it substance. Just as an actor practices for a new role, so too do we need to rehearse new roles.

Affirmations are positive, written statements that, like visualizations, assume a reality that does not yet exist. Remember the exercise of writing forgivenesses in Step 4. Affirmations work in the same way: you construct a sentence and write it twenty times a day. Repeating the statement of intention helps you internalize, and subsequently act on, the affirmation. You signal through nonverbal cues—appearance, posture, walk—as well as through your words and actions how you see yourself. Once you have absorbed a new image of yourself, you present yourself differently to the world, and others respond accordingly.

If you have trouble believing you can actually make one of the changes you saw in your visualization, start with that change. For example, if you let other people take advantage of you and would like to be more assertive, use the following sentence:

> I, Karen, am an assertive person, and I know how to take care of myself.

If you feel awkward in social situations and would like to have more friends, write:

> I, Teresa, have many friends because I am at ease socially.

Write the sentence, or some variation of it, every day until it becomes part of you.

If you have not tried visualizations or affirmations, they may sound like simple wishful thinking to you, but in fact, they can and do work for many people. Our minds and our beliefs about ourselves are powerful determinants of the way we present ourselves to and conduct ourselves in the world. Take yourself seriously: your feelings, your thoughts, your needs. When you do, other people will as well.

BUILDING A LIFE

One of the most important things you can do, must do if you want to move beyond the loss and disappointment of childlessness, is make the commitment to build a worthwhile life for yourself, assuming you do not have one already. *The women who most successfully resolve the loss of childlessness are those who build satisfying and interesting lives.* All the women I talked to who were well along with resolution emphasized the importance of investing in themselves and their lives. This is what they have to say:

- "You have to close the door on having children and open other doors. You have to venture and try as many new experiences as possible."
- "You can't live your life wanting somebody or something to come along and rescue you. You have to be ready for the adventure."
- "You deserve the same things emotionally and materially that people with children and/or spouses have. Don't deprive yourself of a home or wonderful vacations just because your life didn't follow the mainstream."
- "Don't be tied to the dictates of society in your mind. You are still a worthy woman whether you have children or not. Step up and take a wider view. Give yourself a break."
- "Life is not preplanned. There are so many different alternatives out there. But everyone has to feel fulfilled; everyone has to have some outlet for her talent."
- "Your life is your life. Fill it with things that are important to you, things that are interesting to you."

- "You have to make the best of life in the moment. It helps to focus on the positive aspects, the blessings you do have."

The book *Playing Ball on Running Water* by David K. Reynolds, Ph.D., is a helpful guide to living life fully. This book emphasizes the importance of *action and behavior* as contrasted with *feeling and thought*. It is what we *do*, not what we think of doing or what we feel like doing, that will change our lives.

In the beginning, when we first face our childlessness, we may wonder if it will haunt us the rest of our days. It need not. Given time, most women do move beyond the loss.

"I Am Truly Blessed"

ALLISON'S STORY

Allison, a homemaker who is now fifty-two, was a nun for sixteen years. Three years after she left the convent, she met the man who is now her husband. Allison longed to have children, but an early menopause brought her biological time clock to an abrupt end.

"Though I have sadness for the missed experience, I am a full, whole, complete human being. I won't let go of that in trade for anything. Childlessness is not the end of my world. A woman's value is not predicated on the number of children she bears.

"I think the gift I gave myself, the years of commitment to my therapy and my own health, are what have taught me to live with the loss and pain, as we all must learn to do. I learned how to reach inside me for strength I never knew I had. Spirituality is very important in my life. I strive always to be in touch with my own spiritual nature, and I try to relate to the spirit in other people too.

"I would tell a woman facing childlessness that the best sculptor is the one who can take the roughest clay and make something beautiful from it. Confident, creative people are not formed by being handed the life they want on a silver platter. They have to reach deep inside to tap their spiritual strength and their awareness that they control their lives. That is the way they create a beautiful sculpture of their lives.

"Finally, at fifty-two, I can say that I am thrilled to be alive. I enjoy nature and all the beauty and gifts within it. I am satisfied to be with butterflies and rainbows, although I also happily parent any child that comes my way. I am fortunate to live where I do, in the middle of a beautiful desert, with an eleven-thousand-foot mountain in my backyard. Just the other night, I gazed at the sparkling sky, the Milky Way galaxy, and flashing lightning in the distant horizon, and my heart leapt with joy. I thought, 'I am truly blessed.' "

All of us have known sorrow and uncertainty, and we can learn from Allison's story. Because she embraced the quest for feminine wholeness, because she made a commitment to herself and her life, she now knows herself to be a valuable, complete human being. She enjoys the beauty of the world, and she is at peace with herself. She is thrilled to be alive.

"Home to Myself"

ELIZABETH'S STORY

We heard from Elizabeth in Part II when she shared the deeply troubling experience of learning as an adolescent that she was infertile. Now we hear about her resolution process and her quest for wholeness.

"I am only beginning to learn through a long process of psychotherapy how to understand my own history and what effect infertility has had on me. The answers are changing and growing as I do. I felt for so long that my childlessness was somehow *deserved,* that I had no right to a child. I don't feel *that* anymore, but sometimes now I don't even know *what* I feel. I am beginning to have some confidence that I can find out, however.

"To become comfortable with children and to have them love me back has been a healer of my own feelings of inadequacy. I used to feel in some part of my being that children would run from me, but I know now that I am good with them, and that they can love me as I love them. Recently, when my nephew put his arms around my neck and whispered, 'Aunt Elizabeth, next to mommy and daddy I love you best of all,' I was touched to the core. I believe it's important not to deprive yourself of the company of children, thinking that it will be too painful. It is painful, but it is healing and life-giving, too.

"I have a strong spiritual value system and a social conscience that give me a sense of moral well-being. I try to live in such a way that there is an evolution of my loving spirit that benefits me and others. I am able to take pleasure in the beauty of the world and the good things that happen every day.

"Being a feminist is a great boon for me. I cannot easily tolerate any other way of seeing myself as a woman. Feminist literature has helped me gain new perspectives on what it is to be a woman. It has helped me form new beliefs.

"I think I would advise a younger woman who is having trouble coping to be gentle and patient with herself. This is what I am learning to do for *my* younger self! And I would advise therapy, because there is no way that this is easy. It just isn't, and never will be. But life is very short, and it would be tragic to waste it chasing an elusive dream.

"I have gone from being a teenager with no hope of having a baby to being a woman without a child, and, in the process, I have felt the deepest sorrow and loss and brokenness, which have finally come to fruition in my adult life and perhaps brought me home to myself, the self that is, after all, whole, and substantial, and real, though childless."

Elizabeth's journey toward resolution has been long and arduous. We see how far she has traveled in her quest for wholeness when we remember that she used to feel like a deeply flawed person, and now she feels whole and substantial and real. Her story shows that resolution is an ongoing process. Perhaps she, and we, will never arrive at our final destination, but each step along the way is filled with its own rewards.

A LIFELONG QUEST

The quest for feminine wholeness is a lifelong endeavor. As we grow and change, we gain increased understanding of ourselves and others. Our wisdom brings us greater peace, and we find fewer windmills to battle. We appreciate flowers, and rain, and sunsets more than ever before. But balance and harmony are elusive qualities: we find them, only to have them slip away. Now and again, we must pause and refocus:

> to know who we are and what we are and by the knowing find inner peace . . .
>
> to celebrate our spiritual nature, to feel as one with the universe . . .
>
> to honor the wisdom within us, all the while accepting that we continue to learn every day . . .
>
> to appreciate our uniqueness even as we see our relatedness to others . . .

> to live ethically, doing harm to no one and yet taking care of ourselves as well . . .
>
> to strive for personal fulfillment through life's inevitable ebb and flow . . .
>
> to enjoy each day, to feel alive . . .

These are the goals of the quest for wholeness; these are the goals of resolution.

PART FOUR

Starting a Self-Help Group

We all know the tremendous sense of relief and comfort that comes from connecting with another person who has experienced the same traumatic events we have. The more trying our experience—an accident that causes paralysis, a loved one addicted to drugs or alcohol, a child killed by a drunk driver—the more it seems to us that others, even those who are sensitive, caring, and compassionate, cannot really understand our pain and suffering. But when an individual *has* had the same experience, we think, "Yes! She (or he) knows *exactly* what I'm going through!" This immediate sense of shared experience is one of the great strengths of self-help groups.

Self-help groups evolve when people who have similar kinds of problems meet together to help and comfort each other. The groups exist to provide information, support, and peer counseling. As the name suggests, there is usually no professional therapist involved.

Self-help groups validate our feelings and experiences. When other people share what they have been through, we learn that our reactions are not unusual or abnormal. We humans are often hard on ourselves: we blame ourselves for being depressed, for feeling the intense emotions we feel, for not bouncing back immediately. When we see that others also feel depressed or angry, that others do not recover from losses and traumatic events immediately either, we lighten the pressure on ourselves.

We also learn more about ourselves. In the process of trying to explain what it is we think and feel, we clarify our own thoughts and feelings. When we compare ourselves with others in the group, we see that some group members are further along in the healing process than we are, while others have not progressed as far. From those who have progressed further, we learn about the steps that lie ahead; we take hope that the future will be brighter. For those who have not progressed as far, we serve as beacons, and they, in turn, act as signposts to show us how far we have come.

If you can find an existing group for women who will never be mothers, count yourself fortunate. If not, consider starting one. You will not only help yourself; you will help other women as well.

FINDING OTHER WOMEN WHO ARE INTERESTED

If you wish to start a self-help group, you will first need to find other women who are interested in joining. This may not be as difficult as it sounds.

Women you know. When I decided to write this book, I made a list of all the women I knew personally who did not have children. It was a long list. I did not know if some of them had chosen *not* to have children, but I thought that most would have wanted to be mothers. Not all the women I approached agreed to be interviewed, but most did. If you make a list of all the childless women you know, you will probably find many women in your own circle who would be interested in participating in a group.

Word of mouth. I can attest to the fact that almost everyone knows someone who is childless. Wherever I am—the bank, the doctor's office, social occasions—when people learn I am writing a book about women who wanted to be mothers, they say, "Oh, yes, my sister (daughter, cousin, neighbor, colleague) really wanted to have a child and couldn't," or "I know how hard it is because I have a friend who . . ." Tell people you know that you are starting a group and ask if they know anyone who might be interested. No doubt you will find some members this way.

Women's bookstores. Visit women's bookstores in person and talk to the people who work there. Make up fliers and ask if you can leave copies and/or post one on the bulletin board.

Local alternative newspapers. Interest an editor in writing a feature article on the group you plan to start, or place a notice in the classified ads. I did the latter when I wanted to locate women to interview, and I received many responses.

Gynecologists' offices. Start with your own gynecologist but also get the names of infertility specialists in your area. Talk to the staff and leave fliers in the waiting room or post one on the bulletin board.

Women's resource centers. Many universities have women's resource centers, which serve as a central meeting place for women. The center's newsletter informs a wide audience of the various groups available.

PRACTICAL MATTERS

Once you find women who are interested in forming a group, the members will need to make decisions about the following possibilities. There are no right or wrong choices, but it does make sense for the members to discuss and decide, rather than allowing the group to drift. No decisions should be carved in stone; changes can always be made as appropriate.

Leader or no leader? You may want to have a rotating leader for the group. Groups often spend a lot of valuable time just chatting; a leader can help everyone focus and get down to "business." She can also intervene if one or more members dominate the conversation. It is easier and it seems less rude for one person who has designated authority to interrupt a "talker" and redirect the discussion to include others.

If members do decide to have a leader, remember that self-help groups benefit from peer counseling: the leader is *not* expected to be a therapist. In therapy groups, members seek out an expert because they have problems with which they want help. The therapist is accorded a position of greater power and status than other group members because of her expertise. But the leader of a self-help group is *not* expected to set herself apart from the others; her function is one of management.

Where to meet. Groups may meet at members' homes, alternating homes each meeting, or they may meet in neutral territory. Homes provide a warmer, more intimate setting, but some members may not wish to have others come to their homes, or they may be unable to accommodate a large group. If you prefer a neutral setting, many libraries and churches have rooms available for public use free of charge or for a modest fee.

How often to meet. The more often you meet, the more quickly the group will bond together. You may find it difficult to maintain a sense of continuity, especially in the beginning, if you meet infrequently, say, only once a month. However, most people lead such busy lives that a weekly meeting may be inconvenient.

How long to meet. The size of the group will determine to some extent how long the meeting should last. If you have more than three or four members, an hour will probably not be long enough. Even with a large group, two hours may be too long, however. People in groups and therapy sessions tend to avoid sensitive issues, focusing instead on nonthreatening topics, until the session is nearly over. Then there is a rush to deal with the issues they really need to talk about. If you allow too much time, you may find you are wasting much of it.

Open or closed group? Once a group is formed, you will have to decide if new members will be allowed to join or if the membership is closed. New members bring fresh energy and revitalize a group, but they also disrupt, for a time, the established group cohesion and equilibrium. Although there is no ideal group size, two or three members may be too small because of the impact when one member is absent. If the group is large, say, ten to twelve members, there may not be sufficient time for everyone who needs and wants to talk.

Ongoing or limited? Groups can decide to meet a limited number of times, say, ten or twelve, or they can decide to go on indefinitely, as long as members feel they are benefiting. A group that serves its purpose will have some natural attrition as members move toward resolution. For this reason, an ongoing group usually does better if new members are allowed to join.

Refreshments. Refreshments can soften the awkwardness members feel initially and help the members warm up informally. Since many people use food and beverages to comfort themselves, refreshments can also provide reassurance to people who are anxious. If you decide to have refreshments, members can take turns providing them, everyone can bring her own, or one volunteer can bring refreshments and be reimbursed by the others. Alcohol, even wine, should not be available. Alcohol dulls the senses and alters moods, both of which are counterproductive in this kind of setting.

Group Dynamics

Confidentiality

No woman will freely open her heart, talk about her innermost feelings, or make herself vulnerable unless she is certain that what she shares will stay within the group. *Confidentiality will have to be agreed upon by all group members.*

However, my experience with groups has led me to the conclusion that, because the group is meaningful to them, members need and want to share what goes on with significant others in their lives. One way to protect confidentiality *and* allow sharing with others is to agree that no one will divulge names, occupations, or specific identifying information. Instead of saying, "Patricia Ellington who works at the post office told us that . . . ," members can say, "One woman in the group told us that . . ."

Whatever you decide, a clear understanding and firm agreement about confidentiality should be reached in the early stages.

Nonverbal Participants

People who feel shy and inhibited in a group setting may prefer, given a choice, not to talk about themselves at all. Even if members decide, as they probably will, that each woman is expected to share information and feelings about her childlessness, allowances should be made for individual differences. Some people are helped by telling and talking; others are helped by listening and absorbing, in other words, by nonverbal participation.

Personal Responsibility

Group members should be careful about pressuring an individual to expose feelings prematurely. Helping a woman open up her deepest feelings may seem helpful at the time, but it can do more harm than good if the woman is not ready. During the meeting, enormous amounts of support and understanding may be available, but when the individual goes home, she may have no support, no forum to deal with sensitive feelings that have been uncovered. If a group is going to be helpful, members must feel safe. *Each woman must know that she can decide when and how to deal with her own issues.*

Groups work best when members are clear about responsibility. Each member must be responsible for herself: for her own resolution, for getting what she needs from the group. No one, even with the best of intentions, can, or should, decide what someone else needs to do. Excessive focus on others is one way to avoid your own issues.

Avoid labeling, name calling, and diagnosing. They are not helpful! You may—you probably will—have opinions about others, and while it is important to be honest, *how* a thing is said makes all the difference. Instead of saying, "You're denying, you're rationalizing," an approach that will put the other person on the defensive, try tuning in to the feelings you hear behind the words. In a sensitive, caring manner say, "It sounds like you feel . . ." Remember that the group exists to offer support.

Self-help groups have much to offer. In the past few decades they have burgeoned because they have proven themselves to be one of *the most effective* avenues to change for individuals with personal problems. Group support is a powerful force. When we know we are not alone, we find strength to face our inner fears, strength to heal our heartaches. We find courage to build better lives.

Bibliography

Burgwyn, Diana. *Marriage Without Children.* New York: Harper Colophon Books, Harper & Row, 1981.

Eagle, Brooke Medicine. In Jane English, *Childlessness Transformed: Stories of Alternative Parenting.* Mount Shasta, CA: Earth Heart, 1989.

Fallaci, Oriana. *Letter to a Child Never Born.* New York: Simon & Schuster, 1975.

Flinn, Teri. "Taps in the Cabbage Patch." In Ellen Sarasohn Glazer and Susan Lewis Cooper, *Without Child: Experiencing and Resolving Infertility.* Lexington, MA: Lexington Books, 1988.

Frankl, Viktor E. *Man's Search for Meaning.* New York: Simon & Schuster, 1959.

Gibran, Kahlil. *The Prophet.* New York: Knopf, 1979.

Kushner, Harold S. *When Bad Things Happen to Good People.* New York: Avon, 1981.

Lerner, Harriet Goldhor. *Women in Therapy.* Northvale, NJ: Jason Aronson, 1988.

Love, Vicky. *Childless Is Not Less.* Minneapolis, MN: Bethany House, 1984.

Miller, Jean Baker. *Toward a New Psychology of Women.* Boston: Beacon Press, 1986.

Pies, Cheri. *Considering Parenthood: A Workbook for Lesbians.* San Francisco: Spinsters/Aunt Lute, 1985.

Reynolds, David K. *Playing Ball on Running Water.* New York: Quill, 1984.

Sher, Barbara, with Annie Gottlieb. *Wishcraft: How to Get What You Really Want.* New York: Ballantine, 1979.

Stigger, Judith A. *Coping with Infertility: A Guide for Couples, Families, and Counselors.* Minneapolis, MN: Augsburg, 1983.

Questionnaire

Thank you for your willingness to participate in this study. I am a social worker who is gathering material for a book on the subject of childless women who wanted children. Childlessness touches many women, yet receives little attention. I hope through this book to give voice to the disappointment, grief, and resolution that many childless women experience. Any information you share will be strictly confidential. All names and identifying characteristics will be changed in the book.

I want to hear in your own words what being childless has been like and is like for you. Not every question will apply to you, and not every question must be answered.

YOUR BASIC SITUATION NOW

Age. Education. Employment. Marital status. With whom living. Health. Activities you enjoy. Social life. Satisfaction with your life in general. Anything else you think is important.

YOUR EARLY EXPERIENCES AND INFLUENCES

Where did you grow up?

How many children were in your family?

What kind of relationship did you have with your mother? Your father? Your grandparents?

YOUR WISH TO BE A MOTHER

What were your early dreams of having children?

Did you always assume you would be a mother?

What did it mean to you to have a child?

How badly did you want a child?

BEING CHILDLESS

How did it happen that you did not have a child?

What was that like for you?

What feelings do you have about being childless? Are the feelings deep and lingering or passing?

What is/was the hardest part for you?

How did you cope?

Did you talk to others about what you were experiencing?

What helped you resolve the issue, if you have?

SOCIAL ASPECTS

Did/do you feel pressure from others about being childless?

Did you blame yourself? Others? Did you get blamed?

Do you feel there is a social stigma about being childless?

How do you handle the question, "Do you have children?"

If married or in a partnership, did your spouse or partner want children?

Was religion an important factor for you?

Did you think of adopting?

YOUR PRESENT EXPERIENCE

And now, looking back?

Do you still have a sense of loss?

What do you think you have missed?

Are you glad now (sometimes? always?) that you are childless?

What are the compensations, if any, of being childless?

What advice would you give to a younger woman who faces unwanted childlessness and is having trouble coping?

If you could condense into one sentence your feelings about being a woman without a child, what would that sentence be?

Thank you again for sharing. Your help is greatly appreciated.

Index